HORSE MASSAGE
FOR HORSE OWNERS

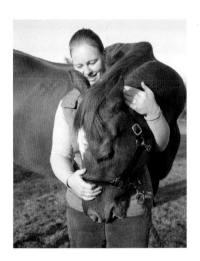

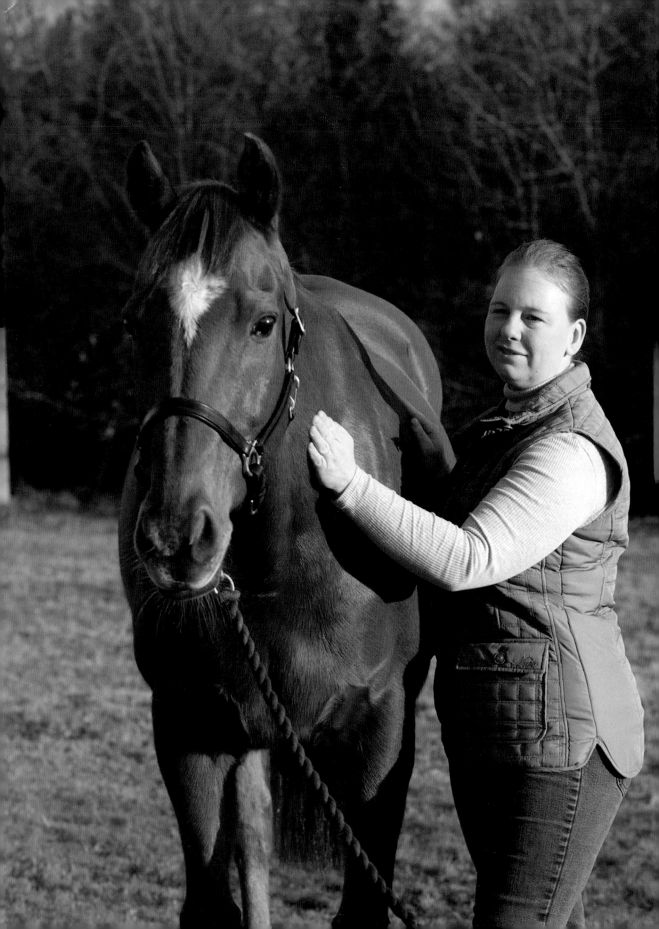

HORSE MASSAGE
FOR HORSE OWNERS
Improve Your Horse's Health and Wellbeing

SUE PALMER

CHARTERED VETERINARY PHYSIOTHERAPIST

J. A. ALLEN · LONDON

First published in Great Britain in 2012 by
J. A. Allen
Clerkenwell House
Clerkenwell Green
London ECIR OHT

J.A. Allen is an imprint of Robert Hale Limited
www.allenbooks.co.uk

ISBN 978-0-85131-999-5

British Library Cataloguing in Publication Data
A catalogue record for this book is available from the British Library

Design and typesetting by Paul Saunders
Edited by Martin Diggle
Line illustrations in Chapter 2 by Samantha Elmhurst BA Hons
Photographs and other images by Simon Palmer,
Into The Lens, except where credited

Printed in Singapore

Disclaimer of Liability

Contents

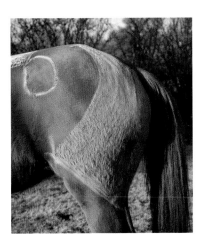
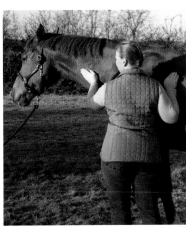
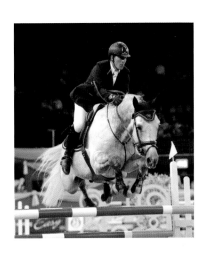

Foreword by **Kelly Marks**

I FIRST MET SUE PALMER (then Sue Brown) over fourteen years ago when she attended one of my Intelligent Horsemanship courses. Sue not only stayed strongly in touch with me – she also married a fellow student, photographer Simon Palmer! I remember Sue's father's wedding speech when he talked about her endless quest for learning and I can vouch for that. Sue has not only studied on my courses and gone on, in fact, to represent us as an Intelligent Horsemanship Recommended Associate, she also went on to study for seven years to qualify as an equine massage therapist and Chartered Veterinary Physiotherapist.

Sue continues to be on a quest for never-ending improvement in horsemanship. She is a fantastic example to anyone who truly wants to do their best for horses in general, or simply for their own much-loved horse. The need to have your horse physically comfortable cannot be overestimated when it comes to his quality of life, and my own horses have regular treatments from Sue. The owner's desire and ability to pay attention to what's happening with their horse, and further, through this book being able to massage him themselves on a regular basis, is an essential element of the respect and understanding that leads to a healthy, happy horse.

Kelly Marks
Intelligent Horsemanship

Preface

MASSAGE HAS BEEN A PASSION for me as long as I can remember, and my objective is that this book will excite a similar passion in you, the reader. My enthusiasm for massage developed over many years. I was lucky enough to be brought up with horses, and have ridden since I was 3 years old. My ponies carried me safely from lead-rein through Pony Club and on to horses, including competing in affiliated showjumping and eventing.

Deciding initially that university wasn't for me, I followed my love of horses through a variety of jobs, working with a range of breeds from Shetland to Shire, and in diverse areas such as driving and point-to-pointing as well as dressage, showjumping, eventing, hacking and teaching. At one time I had my point-to-point jockey's licence, but unfortunately the horse 'did a leg' the week before I was due to ride in my first race, and by the next season racing wasn't an option.

The majority of my time in my late teens and early twenties was spent with a horse dealer. We visited horse fairs including Appleby, Stowe, and Ballinasloe, and were regulars at Southall and Reading Markets. I met horses from all walks of life, including a spell of selling to the knacker-man, and importing top-quality showjumpers from abroad. It was a steep learning curve, one that not many people have the opportunity to experience, and one for which I am forever grateful – I truly believe that I would not be where I am now without the knowledge that I gained during that time.

The horses were my teachers, and those at the dealer's yard taught me far more than any book, DVD, or instructor could ever teach. I learned

Most of my time in late teens and early twenties was spent with a horse dealer.

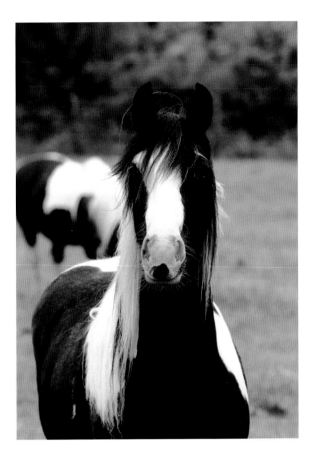

very quickly to assess accurately a horse's behaviour, both on the ground and ridden, because if I got it wrong then I got hurt – which happened on many occasions.

One thing I quickly learned to assess was whether or not a horse had been 'broken-in', and what his ridden behaviour might be. This wasn't something I was conscious of learning, it just 'happened'. I now know that I must have been assessing not only behaviour and attitude, but also muscle tone, reactivity and comfort levels; there was no doubting when I got my assessment wrong – I ended up on the floor!

We had hundreds of unbacked youngsters over the years, either home-bred or bought from the sales, and it was part of my job to back them and prepare them for life in a private home. Many were straight-forward, calmly accepting saddle, bridle and rider in no time at all. Some were more difficult, perhaps more spooky, difficult to get the bridle on, or over-reactive when the girth was done up.

When it was time to move on, I studied hard to qualify and teach as a BHSAI. Around this time a dear friend of mine took me to see a gentleman called Monty Roberts doing a demonstration at Addington Equestrian Centre in Buckinghamshire. I was fascinated, and I remember commenting that it would be a dream come true to study his methods on the course that was then run at West Oxfordshire College. I am a great believer in following your dreams, and so I applied and was accepted to study for the Monty Roberts Preliminary Certificate in Horsemanship with Kelly Marks. In due course I qualified as an Intelligent Horsemanship Recommended Associate (see the Useful Information section near the end of this book for more information), and the behavioural knowledge that I have gained from this work forms an essential part of my massage and physiotherapy work. How else can you persuade a horse to accept the discomfort that physiotherapy sometimes involves, without understanding his behaviour and working *with* him rather than against him? Owners are regularly surprised at how accepting the horse is of the work that I and many other practitioners do, and I'm sure it's because

A friend of mine took me to see a Monty Roberts demonstration in 1997.

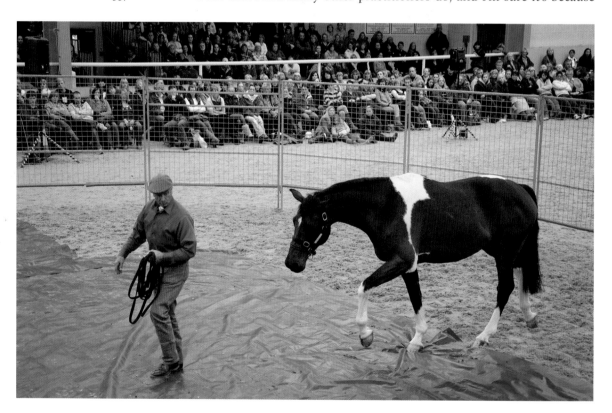

we communicate with the horse, which importantly includes listening to him. At the time of writing, I am the physiotherapist on tour with Monty Roberts and Kelly Marks in the UK, and have been a member of the 'tour team' for several years.

It was when I was teaching riding at Summer Camp in Maine, USA, that I applied to study physiotherapy at university. I was accepted at King's College in London and spent three years studying hard to achieve my BSc, whilst keeping up the horse work to pay the bills. My aim was always to study further to do physiotherapy for horses, but to my surprise I enjoyed working with people so much that I almost changed my mind! The restrictions of employment didn't suit me though; I had spent too many years setting my own hours, and so thankfully I returned to the horses and being self-employed.

I also followed my passion to study massage, initially taking an ITEC diploma in anatomy, physiology and massage, so that I could treat family and friends. Whilst I was at King's College studying physiotherapy, I wanted to understand massage in more depth and to apply more advanced techniques, so I also studied for a qualification in sports massage (ITEC diploma). I took this further to study horse massage with Equinology (see the Useful Infomation section near the end of this book for more information), and qualified as an Equinology Equine Body Worker before studying at the Royal Veterinary College to gain my MSc in veterinary physiotherapy

My work with horses has developed over the years to take into account my knowledge, experience, and the various qualifications as they have progressed. For many years now I have worked freelance to help horses and their owners, whether the issue is caused by 'brain' or 'pain'. With over thirty years of experience, I offer a variety of physiotherapy and teaching techniques including individual and group sessions, courses, demonstrations, and the *Horse Massage for Horse Owners* DVD, first released in 2010. From a routine 'back check', to solving loading issues, to teaching the *Horse Massage for Horse Owners* course, I try to look at the whole picture to support the client towards achieving their dreams with their horse.

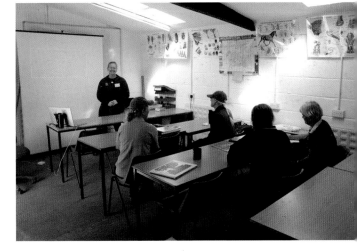

I offer a variety of physiotherapy and teaching options.

I have also contributed to a wide variety of magazines and produce a weekly 'Brain or Pain' e-newsletter giving top tips for equine health and behaviour which you can sign up to from the homepage of my website (www.holistichorsehelp.com), and also a monthly e-magazine, and enjoy maintaining a friendly and supportive Facebook group 'Holistic Horse Help'. I have been overwhelmed by the positive response to the DVD and these other forms of communication, which have allowed me to touch the lives of far more horses than I could ever have hoped to make a difference to, and I hope this book will add to this process.

The combination of a wide variety of experience, traditional qualifications, behavioural qualifications and physical therapy qualifications allows me to offer a holistic approach to working with you and your horse, and in this book I aim to involve you in this approach. Massaging your horse regularly will mean that you can understand him better. The communication between you and your horse will improve as he realises that you are listening to him as much as he tries to listen to you. Through this and the well-documented physical benefits of massage, his health and wellbeing will be enhanced and his performance will improve. And, best of all, massage is something that will be enjoyed by both you and your horse!

Acknowledgements

THIS BOOK IS WRITTEN FOR ALL THE HORSES of the world, and for my very good friend Jo. It could not have been finished without the support of my husband, family, friends and clients, and the patience of the thousands of horses I've learned from.

Thankfully my parents encouraged my passion for horses, and they continue to be there for me, including proof-reading the early versions of this book – thanks mum and dad!

An important person in helping me to be where I am now is Vera Lacey, who took me to my first Monty Roberts demonstration. This ultimately led to working closely with Kelly Marks and Monty Roberts, who continue to provide outstanding inspiration and education, and with the Intelligent Horsemanship Association.

My husband, Simon, was instrumental in filming, editing and producing the *Horse Massage for Horse Owners* DVD that I'm so proud of, and which allowed us to showcase the potential for this book. Crucially, I'd like to thank the many attendees of the Horse Massage for Horse Owners courses, who continued to question, comment, persuade and enthuse until I agreed to put the contents of the course into a format they could take to the yard with them! I am especially appreciative that I was chosen several years ago as the carer of Carol and Don Brazier's stunning black Shire x Thoroughbred Belvedere, who is incredibly tolerant of my ongoing efforts to perfect new techniques, and is the star of my DVD.

My husband also took the photographs in this book, and I thank him for his patience each time I asked for yet another review of the pictures!

We're also grateful to my sister Charlotte for being willing to get very cold posing for massage photographs in the winter, and to Alison Tyler with Spider, owned by the Thoroughbred Rehabilitation Centre, for being such stunning and patient models.

Thanks to Andy White, with his company WowMe! Design, who kindly put together at short notice the diagram that you'll use as a quick reminder of the massage routine. Also thanks to Samantha Elmhurst for the muscle illustrations in Chapter 2, and to Jackie Locheff (www. equimazeequinethermography.co.uk) for use of the image on page 93.

I'd also like to thank Lesley Gowers from J. A. Allen for believing in this current project and getting it off the ground.

Finally, I am eternally grateful for this opportunity to make a difference to the comfort of horses throughout the world, and so I thank anyone and everyone who has helped in any way. Happy massaging!

Introduction

THINK OF THIS BOOK LIKE A RECIPE BOOK. The ingredients of massage are explained and taught separately – anatomy and technique – and then mixed together in specific measures in a specific order with specific timing to create a simple, effective, enjoyable massage routine.

This introduction gives you some background on massage. It is therefore important to read through it, and I ask that you take a few minutes to do so. It will help you to understand what massage is, and why I recommend that you massage your horse on a regular basis. I believe that you will be far more motivated to massage your horse regularly if you understand why you are doing so.

The first chapter, Learning Massage, is where we start getting practical. You will learn initially to massage using yourself as the subject (your forearm) and/or a friend or partner. This gives you the chance to make mistakes without worrying about the consequences, to receive valuable feedback on how well you're doing, and to sharpen your skills until you feel you're ready to take them to your horse.

The second chapter, Equine Anatomy, explains *where* you will be massaging, and why it's important to massage there. The anatomy of the horse is fascinating and incredible. Built for both speed and endurance, a complex system of bones, ligaments, tendons and muscles comprises

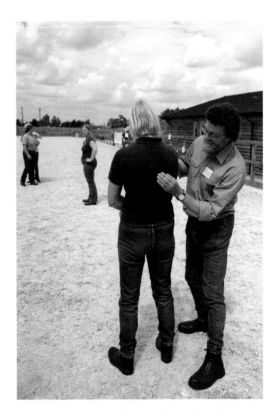

In Chapter 1 Learning Massage you learn the massage techniques using yourself or a partner as the subject, giving you the chance to make mistakes without worrying about the consequences.

the musculoskeletal system that you will be working with. This might sound complicated but you needn't worry, I've chosen seven key muscles to discuss (I'm counting the pectoral group as one here – see Chapter 2) and, through an awareness of these, you will be able to create an effect throughout the entire body.

Chapter 3, Massaging Your Horse, pulls together all the information given so far and puts it into a full body massage routine for you to use with your own horse. I'm hoping that you will take this book to the yard with you as a reference, and you will be able to look at it to remind yourself of anything you're unsure of. At the back of the book is a useful 'prompt section' to help you remember the routine described in Chapter 3.

Chapter 4, Problem-solving, focuses on common training issues and behavioural problems that I see on a regular basis, and how you might be able to help overcome some of these using massage. This chapter aims to help you to help your horse, in an effort to reduce stiffness and pain and to improve performance. *It is not intended to replace the advice of a qualified professional.*

Chapter 4 Problem-solving focuses on helping you to overcome common training issues with your horse through massage.

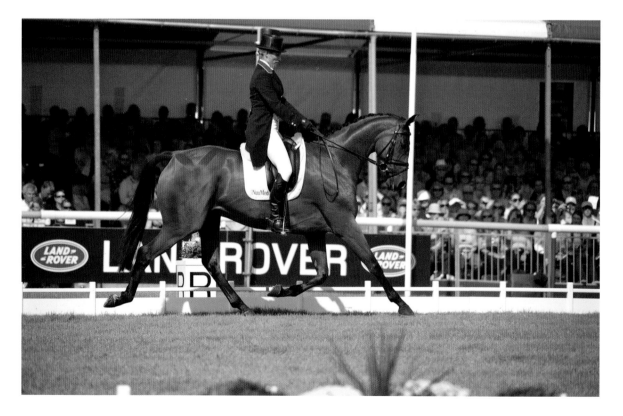

Chapter 5, Frequently Asked Questions, does exactly what it says on the tin. I have been teaching the Horse Massage for Horse Owners course for several years now, and there are certain questions that come up every time. I've included these in this chapter in the hope that I will cover the majority of your questions, along with providing some useful background information.

The final Useful Information section offers advice on where to go for further information. Often you will find that one interesting link will lead you to another, and so on, enabling you to personalise your learning to suit you and your horse, and to continue to improve your knowledge and skills.

There are many different schools of massage, and many different approaches to equine therapy. This book is written from my own viewpoint (excepting the anatomy information, which is universal). There are, of course, some areas where there is no confusion or ambiguity, but massage in general is open to interpretation, both in the equine and the human field. This text is intended to give you the confidence to get started, to put your hands on your horse and 'give it a go'. If it achieves this goal then I have succeeded in my objective, and I know that your horse will appreciate your efforts. If you want to stick with what you learn in this book, then there is more than enough here for you to be able to give long-term benefit to your horse and, at the same time, enjoy for yourself the advantages that you are giving him. If you are inspired to look into massage or physiotherapy in more detail then I would encourage that, and there is plenty to look into.

Throughout this book I refer to your horse as 'he'. This is to reduce the number of times I need to write 'he or she', and because I can't bear horses being referred to as 'it'. Please accept my apologies if your horse is a mare, and understand my reasoning behind this decision!

Aims and objectives

WHAT THIS BOOK WILL DO FOR YOU

This book will teach you a basic massage routine that you can practise on your own horse. It is written as an introduction to massage, and if you would like to learn more there are numerous excellent books and courses available throughout the world. Massaging your horse regularly will help you to detect earlier whether there might be physical issues or problems with your horse's musculature. Through increasing your awareness of what is normal for your horse, you will be better able to recognise what is not normal. Regular massage will also enable you to promote your horse's health and wellbeing actively. I've been told countless times that owners have experienced the best work from their horse when they've massaged him beforehand. You will be able to massage your horse in between visits from a professional, so that you're better able to support the work that they do and help maintain your horse between treatments. This book will, of course (and possibly most importantly) offer you a way of spending quality time with your horse, and the ability to give something back to him for all that he has given you.

WHAT THIS BOOK WILL *NOT* DO FOR YOU

Most importantly, this book does not and will not act as a substitute for the advice or therapeutic input of a professional. That includes veterinarians, physiotherapists, osteopaths, chiropractors, massage therapists, and any other paraprofessional who has spent many years learning their trade. This book will not teach you how to fix your horse, although it will enable you more easily to support those whom you employ to work with him. It does not give you a qualification in massage, or qualify you to treat horses. It simply teaches you a routine to use with your own horse. This may sound obvious or strict, but once you read the section in Chapter 5 on the law relating to physiotherapy for animals you will hopefully understand better why I feel the need to state these facts clearly.

What is massage?

'Massage is the practice of applying structured or unstructured pressure, tension, motion, or vibration – manually or with mechanical aids – to the soft tissues of the body, including muscles, connective tissue, tendons, ligaments, joints and lymphatic vessels to achieve a beneficial response.' (*Wikipedia*).

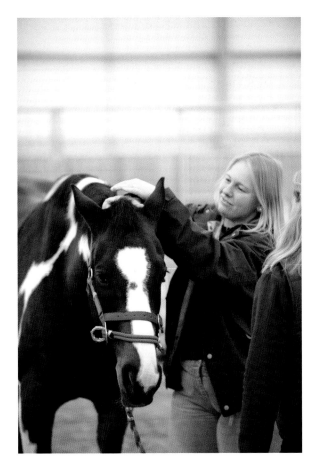

'Massage is the practice of applying structured or unstructured pressure, tension, motion, or vibration – manually or with mechanical aids – to the soft tissues of the body, including muscles, connective tissue, tendons, ligaments, joints and lymphatic vessels to achieve a beneficial response.' (*Wikipedia*)

I particularly like this definition because it covers so much. Take the first part of the sentence, 'massage is the practice of applying structured or unstructured ...' In this book you will learn a very structured approach to massaging your horse. This is because I believe that it's easier to learn initially if you're following clear guidelines. However, massage can be structured or unstructured, and my hope is that once you're confident with the techniques taught here you will start to develop your own massage routine, with or without structure, that is individual to you and your horse.

Massage involves 'pressure, tension, motion or vibration'. Again, I find this useful and thought-provoking. Throughout this book I will talk about using pressure, albeit often very lightly, to massage your horse. There are many ways of describing massage techniques, and many massage techniques to describe. Please bear in mind that the techniques that

I discuss here I have chosen because they suit my purpose of creating confidence in you, the reader, to give a safe and effective massage to your own horse.

Wikipedia goes on to mention that massage can be done manually or with mechanical aids, and this is as relevant in the equine field as it is in the human field. This book teaches you about a manual therapy, using your hands to help your horse. I believe there is something about the healing power of touch that most people are aware of but that has not yet been fully proven by science, and so far cannot be replaced by any machine. Massage allows you to use this potential for the benefit of your horse.

The definition states that massage is applied 'to the soft tissues of the body, including muscles, connective tissue, tendons, ligaments, joints and lymphatic vessels'. This is a great reminder that when we massage our horse, we are having an effect on the whole horse. It is clear from the horses' response that massage affects far more than just the skin and the muscles.

The last part of the definition points out that massage is done 'to achieve a beneficial response'. This is probably my favourite phrase from that descriptive sentence. There are so many reasons you might have for massaging your horse, but all of them can be encompassed in one simple phrase: 'to achieve a beneficial response'.

The massage that you will learn through this book is known as 'Swedish massage' or 'classic massage'. There are five basic strokes in Swedish massage – don't worry if the names of the techniques sound strange, they will be second nature by the time you try them on your horse! The routine you will use with your horse will involve effleurage (stroking), petrissage (compression and kneading), and tapotement (cupping). Chapter 4, Problem-solving, includes the use of friction (cross-fibre friction).

Massage has been around a long time, and is here to stay. It is a manual therapy that can be practised by almost anyone. At its most basic, massage is a simple way of easing pain, while at the same time aiding relaxation and promoting a feeling of wellbeing and a sense of receiving good care. It is something to be enjoyed both by the person massaging and by the person, or horse, being massaged. Once learned, it is a skill for life.

Why massage?

Anyone who has had a massage will tell you that being massaged feels good, and so at the very least (and possibly best of all) you can offer this feeling to your horse.

You might choose to massage your horse simply because you want to offer him something in return for all that he has done for you. We get so much from our horses that it's great to be able to give something back. It might be that you know your horse has a problem, and you want to help him either to overcome this problem, or to manage it more comfortably. You may have regular therapy for your horse, and want to support the work that the therapist does in between treatment sessions.

An older horse will appreciate massage to ease his potentially aching joints. A younger horse will benefit from massage to help him enjoy learning to stand still and accept treatment, which will be of benefit throughout his life. An injured horse, especially one on box rest, will find that massage helps relieve discomfort and maintain suppleness whilst he is unable to exercise fully. A competition horse will find it easier to perform to the best of his ability when he is more comfortable and more flexible, and massage will help him to achieve this. The horse who is in

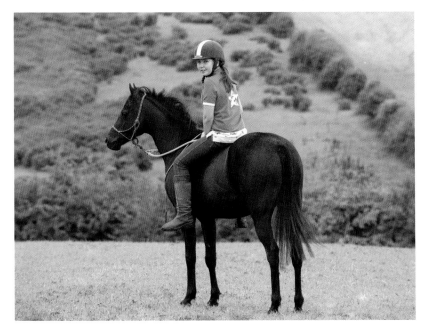

You might choose to massage your horse simply because you want to offer him something in return for all that he has done for you.

A competition horse will find it easier to perform to the best of his ability when he is more comfortable and more flexible, and massage will help him to achieve this.

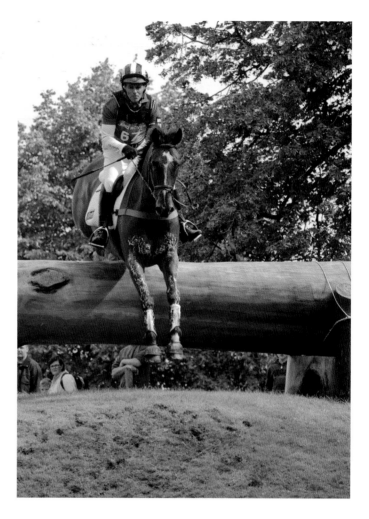

need of support, for example an abused horse, one who is recovering from trauma, a horse who has been passed from home to home, one who is difficult to catch or one who appears to be grieving, will benefit from the love and attention that massage allows you to offer him.

A horse who struggles to work through from behind, or to work through his back, or to relax to the contact, or to bend correctly, or to pick up canter on the correct lead, or to halt square, or to move laterally, could benefit from massage. A horse who often canters disunited, or is reluctant to go forward, who stops at fences, or rushes his fences, who always has a pole down, or struggles to make the distance, could find his performance improved with massage. A horse who naps, or bucks going into canter, or who bites when you do his girth up, or is ticklish

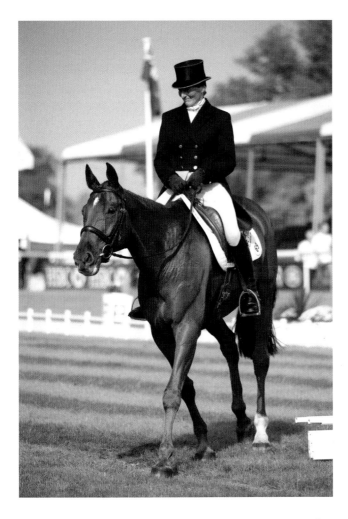

Ridden behaviour and performance might be improved through massage.

to be brushed, who refuses to stand to be saddled or mounted, or rushes off for the first few strides, might find his behaviour improved with massage.

You might travel your horse to competitions where he then needs to stay away from home, and massage could help him to relax and therefore enhance his performance. A horse with difficult behaviour can benefit from massage to encourage him to be more accepting of human demands. I even had one client who used massage to help introduce a difficult young horse to being clipped! There are so many excellent reasons to massage your horse that it's impossible to list them all here, and anyway your purpose will be individual to you and your horse. As long as your intention is good, then massage will be of benefit to your horse.

A short exercise that I use on the Horse Massage for Horse Owners courses to demonstrate to people why they might want to massage their horse is this. Find a space to walk around in, and lock your ankle up tight. Try walking for a minute or two, and see how you feel. Frequent comments are that people feel tight through their leg, sore in their back or neck, tight all up one side of their body, locked up in their shoulder, sore through their hip (on either side); they have a shorter stride with one leg, they are less balanced, less confident, less willing to go forwards, more likely to have an accident. Trying out this exercise will really bring home to you how a problem in just one joint can have a widespread effect on the entire body, resulting in pain and stiffness far from the original problem, and having a strong effect on behaviour. Just imagine being a horse feeling that way, and then having a rider insisting – sometimes violently – that you carry out your work as normal! Think about that the next time you see someone whipping their horse for napping, digging their spurs in as he stops at a fence, tying his head down with training aids to stop difficult behaviour, or yanking him in the mouth when he resists the contact.

Try walking with one ankle held very stiffly, and feel the knock-on effects throughout your body. Imagine a horse who is stiff or sore in his neck, back, hock, fetlock or foot, and how this will have a far-reaching effect, including on his balance and willingness to go forwards.

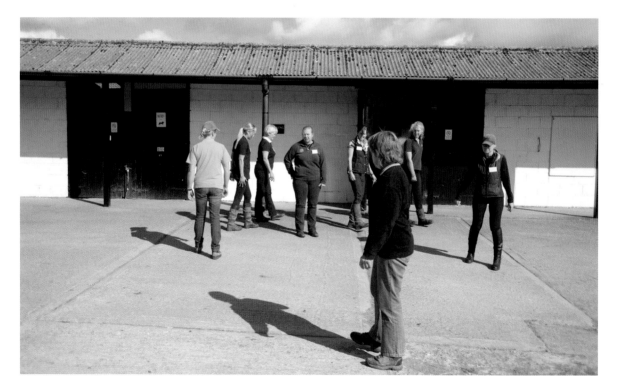

Glossary

I've tried to keep this book as user-friendly as possible and you will find, within the main text, explanations of how the scientific names of the muscles relate to their structure and how this, in turn, relates to their function. However, there are also a few anatomical and directional terms used in the text, explanations of which are listed below for guidance.

Abduct: to move away from the midline of the body

Adduct: to move towards the midline of the body

Caudal: towards the tail

Cervical: relating to the neck

Cranial: towards the skull

Distal: furthest from the point of attachment or centre of the body

Dorsal: towards the back

Lateral: towards the side

Lumbar: relating to the part of the body between the lowest ribs and the pelvic bones

Medial: towards the middle

Proximal: nearest the point of attachment or centre of the body

Sacral: related to the sacrum

Thoracic: relating to the thorax

Ventral: towards the belly

A form of shorthand is used in relation to anatomical terms. In the context of this book, this is especially relevant in terms of the vertebrae of the spine. The capital letter refers to the area of the spine and the number following refers to the relevant vertebra, for example:

C3 is the third cervical vertebra

T3 is the third thoracic vertebra

L3 is the third lumbar vertebra

S3 is the third sacral vertebra

1. Learning Massage

In this chapter you will:

- Learn the massage techniques of effleurage (stroking), petrissage (compression and kneading), tapotement (cupping), and friction (cross-fibre friction).
- Practise these techniques on yourself and on a partner.
- Develop confidence and 'feel' through this practice.
- Recognise and overcome common mistakes in the learning process.

We begin our practical learning on ourselves or on another human being, rather than on a horse. This has several benefits:

- You can learn, understand and remember each move clearly, allowing yourself more time to focus on your breathing and your posture, which are important factors when you are massaging your horse.
- You can practise as many times as you like without your horse getting fidgety.
- You can discover how different the muscle tone and skin stretch feels in different areas (even just the differences from your elbow to your fingertips), and begin to accept these different sensations.
- You can develop a feel for 'normal' muscle tone, and therefore begin to determine what is 'not normal' muscle tone.

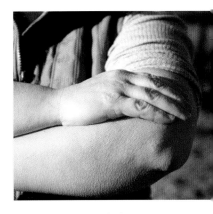

We begin our practical learning on ourselves or on another human being, rather than on a horse.

- You can feel what it's like if you massage over a bony area compared to over a muscular area.

- You can search for 'knots' in the muscle and get feedback as to whether you have found what you think you have found.

- You can make mistakes without upsetting your horse.

- You can practise without needing to be at the stables, and perfect your moves by the time you get to your horse so you can make the most of your time with him.

- You can experiment with working more firmly, more softly, faster or slower, and decide which is most beneficial in your opinion.

- If you have a willing friend or partner, they can try the moves on you, so that you can feel what it's like to be the subject as well as to be the practitioner.

- You can get verbal feedback to let you know how the massage feels (as opposed to physical feedback from teeth or hooves!).

- You can develop confidence in your technique, which in turn will improve your skill level.

Preparation

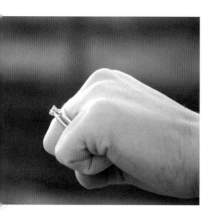

Stones from rings could dig into the skin, potentially causing discomfort and an adverse reaction from your partner or horse.

You can practise these techniques on your own arm, and/or on a friend or partner's back. I recommend that you remove any rings, watches or bracelets, or turn rings over so that stones don't press into the person you are massaging.

If you are practising on your own arm, wear a short-sleeved T-shirt or roll up your sleeves. Your hands need to be dry in order for them to slide smoothly over your skin. I find it's easiest to practise on the upper side of my forearm, working from my wrist towards my elbow. Practising on a partner is discussed later in this chapter.

The ideal is to practise initially on yourself so that you can understand what the techniques feel like, and then practise on a partner to get verbal feedback. Try working faster, slower, and with more or less pressure, and see what the response is. If your partner is willing, ask them to practise the techniques on you as well.

Practising on yourself

Effleurage

Place your hand, palm down, onto your other forearm just above your wrist. Apply a little pressure, mostly through the heel of your hand. Have the whole of the palm of your hand, including the pads of your fingers and thumb, relaxed and in contact with your forearm. Maintaining the same pressure all the way, slide your hand up towards your elbow. You will see the skin ripple slightly in a wave in front of your hand as you move. When your hand is close to your elbow, stop and release the pressure, so that your hand just rests lightly against your forearm again. Without any pressure, but keeping your hand in contact with your arm, slide your hand back down your forearm to just above your wrist, where you started. Repeat this as many times as you need in order to become comfortable with the technique.

I suggest taking around four seconds to slide your hand up from wrist to elbow, and around four seconds to slide back down again.

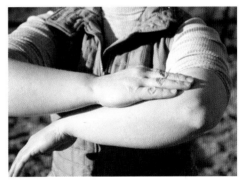

ABOVE Apply effleurage from wrist towards elbow, then release the pressure and slide back to your starting position.

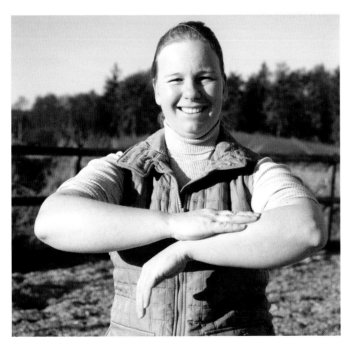

To practise on yourself, start by placing your hand, palm down, onto your forearm just above your wrist.

4 sec

Take around four seconds to slide your hand from wrist to elbow, and around four seconds to slide back down again.

Petrissage: compression

Rest your hand lightly on your other forearm, just above your wrist, and slide it slowly towards your elbow. As you reach the end of your forearm, stop and press the heel of your hand down to squash the muscle it was resting on. Keep the rest of your hand relaxed and in contact with your skin while you do this. Use the heel of your hand to slide your skin up towards your elbow, as far as your skin is able to stretch. This won't be very far so don't expect too much, and it's important that you take the skin *with* your hand, rather than sliding over the top of it. Once you've stretched the skin as far as it will go, slowly and gently release the pressure, and then slide your hand a couple of centimetres back in the direction of your wrist. Repeat the process, first squashing the muscle, then stretching the skin towards your elbow, releasing the pressure, and then sliding your hand a couple of centimetres back towards your wrist to start again in a new spot.

Think of this compression technique as a four-second move. It takes around a second to press into the skin and squash the muscle, around a second to stretch the skin, around a second to release the pressure, and around a second to slide to your next starting point.

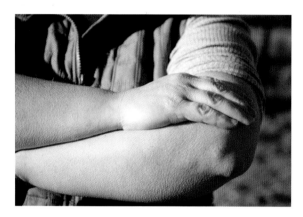

For the compression move, start by sliding your hand towards your elbow. As you reach the end of your forearm, stop and press the heel of your hand down to squash the muscle it was resting on. Then use the heel of your hand to slide your skin up towards your elbow, as far as your skin is able to stretch.

Petrissage: kneading

Make a fist with your hand, and place the flat surface between your knuckles and your finger joints against your skin. Slowly and firmly press into the skin and muscle, squashing it under your hand. Keeping the muscle squashed, gently rotate your wrist and forearm so that the skin under your fist is stretched into a twist. Once the skin has moved as much as it's able to, slowly release the pressure, unwinding your fist and the skin underneath it as you do so, then move a few centimetres to a new area and begin again. Work anywhere between your wrist and your elbow, in no particular pattern.

As with many of the other techniques I describe here, think of kneading as a four-second move. Take around one second to squash the

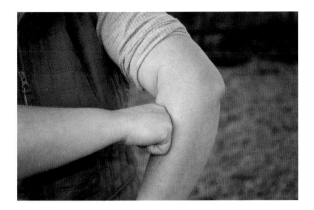

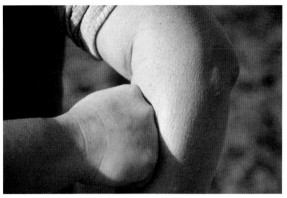

In the kneading move, make a fist with your hand, and place the flat surface between your knuckles and your finger joints against your skin. Slowly and firmly press into the skin and muscle, squashing it under your hand.

Keeping the muscle squashed, gently rotate your arm so that the skin under your fist is stretched into a twist.

skin, around one second to twist the skin, around one second to relax and unwind the skin, and around one second to slide gently to your next spot. As in the compression technique, move slowly and smoothly for maximum comfort and benefit.

Tapotement: cupping

Make a 'cup' from your hand, so that the edges of your hand (including your little finger, the pads of your fingers, your thumb and the heel of your hand) are in contact with your forearm. Softly tap your cupped hand against the muscle on your fore-arm so that you can see a slight wobble through the surrounding areas. Work in a rhythm that suits you, perhaps two to four taps per second.

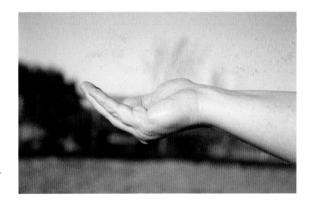

For cupping, make a 'cup' from your hand.

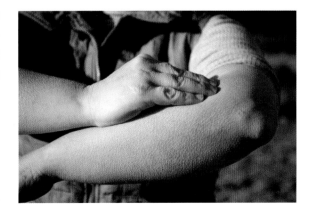

RIGHT Place the edges of your hand (including your little finger, the pads of your fingers, your thumb and the heel of your hand) in contact with your forearm, then softly tap the muscle, working in a rhythm.

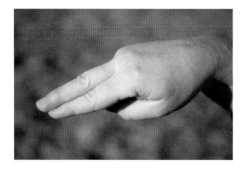

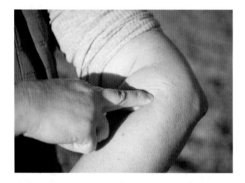

TOP It's important to use two fingers to support each other when you are using this cross-fibre friction technique, or four fingers if you find that more comfortable.

BOTTOM Keeping the muscle squashed, slowly circle the skin, taking it to maximum stretch around the circle.

Cross-fibre friction

Cross-fibre friction is a technique that is not included in the massage routine in this book. However, if you find an area that would benefit from further massage work, it is a great technique to use. I refer to it often in Chapter 4 Problem-solving.

It's important to use two fingers to support each other when you are using this technique. This is to avoid straining and potentially causing injury to the finger that is applying the pressure. With one finger on top of the other, place your fingers on the skin, and squash down into the muscle. Keeping the muscle squashed, slowly circle the skin, taking it to maximum stretch around the circle.

Move slowly to allow the body time to react to the sensation; each circle should take around four seconds to complete. Keep circling until you feel that the skin and muscle have softened under your fingers, then release the pressure and move to another spot.

Practising on a partner

Practising on a partner requires some thought with regards to posture, and where on your partner to apply the techniques. The principles are exactly the same as when you are practising on your forearm. The muscle I recommend working on is the long back muscle that runs either side of the spine, so the first thing you need to do is locate this muscle. It's easiest if your partner wears just a T-shirt or shirt; it can be difficult to feel through thick layers of clothing. Feel between their shoulder-blades and move your fingers from side to side to find their spine. Then ask your partner to put one hand behind their back, and you will see that their shoulder-blade sticks out a little. Feel where the inside of their shoulder-blade is. The long back muscle that you are looking for is the area of the back between the inside of their shoulder-blade and their spine. It runs from the base of their back to the base of their neck, either side of their spine.

Next, you need to think about your own posture if you are practising with a partner. Stand to the side of them, facing at 90 degrees to the

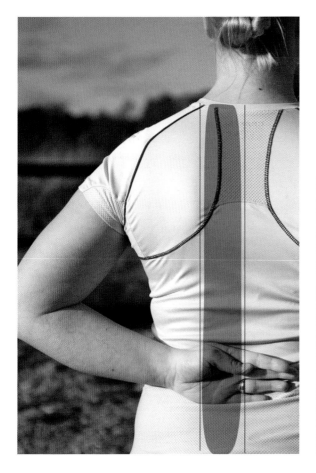

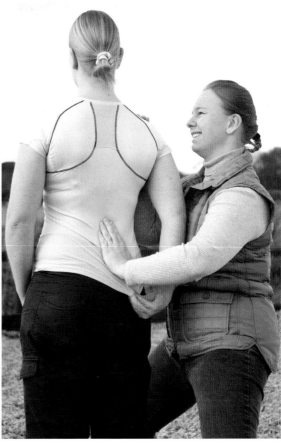

direction that they are facing, with your feet a little apart and your knees slightly bent. Rest one hand on the front of their shoulder, and allow your forearm to rest along the front of their upper arm. This is to provide support to your partner so that they feel balanced when you press on their back. Make sure that your hand rests just lightly on their shoulder, rather than pulling down. Your other hand massages their long back muscle.

If the person you are practising on is taller than you, ask them to stand with their feet apart and their knees bent until their back is at a comfortable height for you to work with. If you are taller than the person that you are practising on, they could stand on a block, or you could move your feet wider apart and bend your knees more. Try to avoid bending from your waist any more than is essential, as this will put strain through your own back, and before long you'll be looking for treatment for yourself!

ABOVE LEFT To find your friend's long back muscle, find their spine and the inside of their shoulder-blade. The muscle between these on either side of the spine running from the base of the back to the base of the neck is the long back muscle.

ABOVE RIGHT If you are practising on a friend, think about your posture. Correct posture will improve not only your own comfort, but also the effectiveness of the massage techniques that you are practising.

You will find that, when you massage up the long back muscle from the base of the back towards the base of the neck, the person's clothing will have a tendency to wrinkle up under your fingers, which prevents you from giving a smooth massage move. To reduce this problem, ask the person to put both hands behind their back and take hold of the bottom of their shirt, pulling it downwards so that it's taut. You'll still be able to feel their back muscle through the shirt, but won't have the interference of the fabric getting in the way of your technique.

If you have the opportunity, try the technique on several different friends. See how their feedback varies and how your confidence improves.

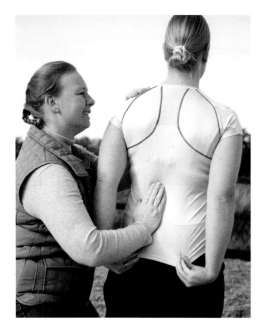

Apply effleurage from base of back towards base of neck, then release the pressure and slide slowly back to your starting position.

To prevent your friend's clothing from wrinkling when you practise your massage techniques, ask them to hold the back of their shirt down.

Effleurage: stroking

Follow the instructions given for practising effleurage on yourself, but begin by placing your hand, palm down, onto the base of your partner's back. Be aware of your posture, and that your free hand rests just lightly on their shoulder with your forearm offering support to the front of their body. Apply pressure as you begin effleurage from the base of the back towards the base of the neck. You will see your partner's clothing ripple slightly in a wave in front of your hand as you move, mirroring what is happening to their skin (it's important that they have pulled their shirt tight so that it doesn't get caught up in front of your fingers). When you are close to their neck, release any pressure and slide your hand down their back again to the point that you started from.

Petrissage: compression

Follow the directions for practising compression on yourself as you learn the technique on your partner. Begin with your hand resting lightly on the base of your partner's back, and slide it slowly towards their neck. Use the compression technique as your hand returns from the base of the neck towards the base of the back. Always stretch the skin *away* from yourself in the compression move, which in this case means you will be stretching the skin *towards* your partner's neck.

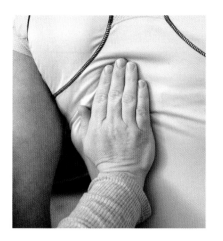

LEFT If you are working with a friend practising the compression technique, use the heel of your hand to stretch their skin, through their clothing, up towards their neck as far as their skin is able to stretch. Remember to ask for verbal feedback and adjust your technique accordingly.

RIGHT In kneading, work anywhere on your partner's lower back, in no particular pattern.

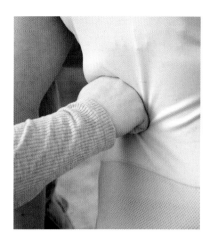

Petrissage: kneading

Being sure to support your partner, make a fist with your hand, and place the flat surface between your knuckles and your finger joints against your partner's clothing on their low back. Practise kneading anywhere on your partner's lower back, in no particular pattern. In most cases, it is not comfortable for you to work between the shoulder-blades, because the width of your fist is wider than the width between the spine and the inside of the shoulder-blade, and therefore you would be massaging over a bony area, which is unpleasant for the person being massaged.

Tapotement: cupping

If your partner is standing up then you will only be able to use one hand, as you can when you practise on yourself. However, if your partner is lying face down for you to practise, you can use both hands, working alternately for the cupping technique, which is what you will do when you massage your horse. You can only use this technique on your partner's lower back because the size of your hand will be too big to use it between the shoulder-blade and the spine.

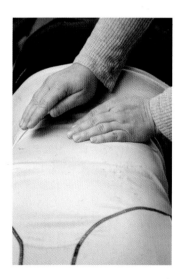

Use both hands for the cupping technique if possible.

Cross-fibre friction

See whether you can find a 'knot' in your partner's muscles. The easiest place is usually around the top of and the inside of the shoulder-blade.

The 'knot' might feel like a bit of grit in the muscle, or like a tiny piece of rope, or like a small pea under the skin. Often you can confirm that it's a knot by applying deep pressure as you move over it, and judging your partner's reaction – if it's a knot then deep pressure may well be painful for them. With one finger on top of the other, practise cross-fibre friction around your partner's shoulder region, using verbal feedback to help you improve your technique.

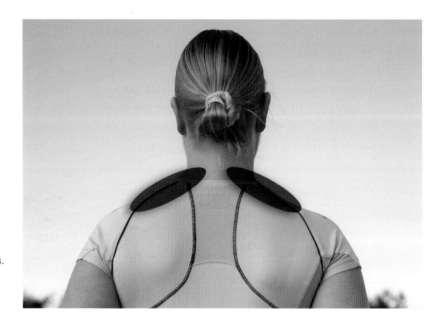

See whether you can find a 'knot' in your partner's muscles. The easiest place is usually around the top and the inside of the shoulder-blade.

Helpful hints

Relax

The most common mistake I see when people are first learning massage is that their fingers are tense, which means that their hand is not relaxed. In effleurage tense fingers mean that the pads of the fingers lose contact with the skin. Try deliberately tensing your fingers so that they lift away from the skin, and notice how different the effleurage feels, both for the giver and for the receiver. Then relax your fingers again and feel how much smoother the contact is, and how much better you are able to feel the tissues that you are massaging.

In the compression technique, it's easy to start pressing into the body with the tips of your fingers. Instead, check that the palm of your hand and the pads of your fingers are lying softly on the skin throughout the move, including when you are stretching the skin towards them. Some people allow the pads of their fingers to slide over the skin as the heel of the hand moves in that direction; others keep the pads of their fingers still, so that the palm of their hand is raised away from the skin during the stretch part of the move. Either technique is fine, as long as there is continual contact and no pressure from anywhere except for the heel of your hand.

When you are practising on a partner, your fingers should be so relaxed that, when you reach the top of their back, your fingers naturally follow the contour of the body and curve over the shoulder. The same applies to massaging the shoulder region of your horse when you reach the withers.

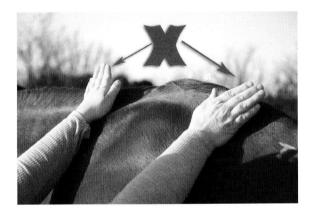 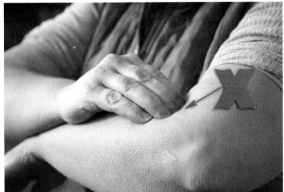

ABOVE LEFT Avoid letting the pads of your fingers lose contact with the skin; this would suggest that your hands are tense and will affect the quality of the massage you offer.

ABOVE RIGHT Check that the palm of your hand and the pads of your fingers are lying softly on the skin throughout the compression move, including when you are stretching the skin towards them.

Slow down

There is a tendency for people to move too fast when they are massaging. They are often unaware of this. I find this problem most common in people who have busy lives, whether with work, family or other commitments. For this reason I've suggested a specific timing for each move. Sometimes people massage in a rough way, instead of smooth and flowing. One of my favourite phrases that I learned from Monty Roberts is to 'move as though you're moving through sticky treacle', and this applies equally as well to massage as it does to handling your horse.

In compression, for example, the tendency (incorrect in this case) can be to push rapidly into the muscle for the first part of the move and then wait a second before the next part. Then the skin is moved quickly, and held for a second before suddenly being released. Another second goes by and then the hand is moved swiftly to the next spot. Instead of this sharp application of the technique, think first about taking a second or so to ease your hand into the skin and let it sink gently into the muscle. Then take around a second to effortlessly encourage the skin to stretch away from you, taking care that your hand moves with the skin and the skin moves with your hand, rather than your hand moving over the skin (or clothing). Think 'slow' as you gradually ease off the pressure until you have the lightest touch, and then glide your hand slowly over the skin to complete the fourth part of the move.

Think seriously about how long four seconds is. It's not just the time it takes you to count to four as quickly as you can! Make sure that, in your cross-fibre friction move, each circle takes around four seconds to complete, allowing the body enough time to react to the stretches and mobilisations that you are applying.

Stay in touch

It's important to keep physical contact at all times with the person or horse you're massaging, including when you are moving from one technique to the next. For example, when you reach the end of your effleurage stroke, it's easy to think that you've done the move and to take your hand away from the body as you go back to the beginning to repeat the move,

Keep your hand in contact with the skin at all times.

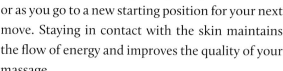

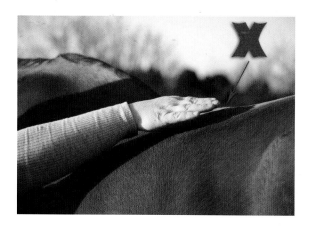

or as you go to a new starting position for your next move. Staying in contact with the skin maintains the flow of energy and improves the quality of your massage.

Master the technique

Often people find it difficult to separate out the four sections of the compression and the kneading moves. Like every massage technique described here, it isn't actually essential to carry out the move in a particular way, since you are unlikely to cause any harm through doing it differently. It is essential, however, to know exactly what your hands are doing, and it's amazing how much we do without being aware of it. This lack of awareness will hamper your ability to assess your horse's health and wellbeing through his musculature. For this reason, I am very specific about how to do each move. Once you have mastered them, and are able to control the speed and direction of your hands, you can adjust the techniques if necessary to suit you and your horse.

Stretch the slack

It's tempting to try to twist further than the skin is able to move in the compression, kneading and cross-fibre friction techniques. Some areas of skin have very little movement. Try using your finger to move the skin on the back of your hand in a circle, and then try the same on the palm of your hand, and notice the difference. There is much more 'skin slack' on the back of your hand, which means that you can cause more movement there. Bear this in mind when you're using these techniques, and only stretch or twist the skin as far as it's able to go. As you work on your own arm, you'll be able to see the stretch through the skin, and the wrinkles you cause where you're working as your skin is 'scrunched up'.

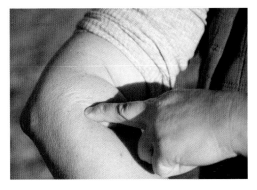

Stretch the skin with your fingers, rather than moving over the skin.

Use a flat fist

If you use the joints that project when you make a fist to carry out this massage technique, it could be very uncomfortable, particularly on areas where you are working close to the bone. Make a fist, and use the flat surface of your fingers rather than your knuckles or the joints in your fingers.

Knead with your wrist straight

Kneading should come from your shoulder and your entire arm, not just from your wrist. The aim is to make a fist with your hand, and keep your wrist as straight as possible to minimise any strain through it. Wrists

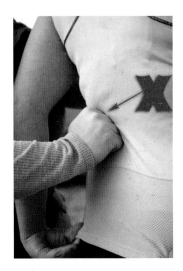

Use the flat surface of your knuckles.

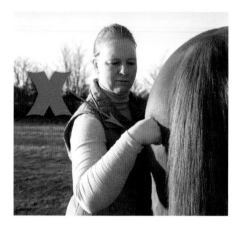 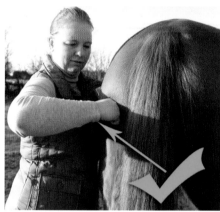

Keep your wrist as straight as possible, to minimise any strain through it.

are prone to repetitive strain injuries, and you could aggravate these if you massage with your wrist flexed during this technique. Depending on where you are massaging, and the height of the person or horse that you're massaging, this means you may need to move your elbow, and even your body.

Cup with both hands

Remember to use both hands for cupping. When you are practising on your partner or working with your horse, alternate your hands, using one then the other. Try to find a comfortable rhythm to work in – you can use the massage on yourself and your partner to experiment with different rhythms. See which feels best for you, and which your partner prefers.

This technique is gentler with the hands cupped rather than flat. Flat hands remind me of 'slapping', which is not nearly so comfortable for the

BELOW LEFT Alternate your hands, using one then the other then the first again, and so on. Find a comfortable rhythm to work in.

BELOW RIGHT Keep your hand cupped.

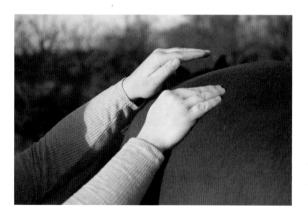 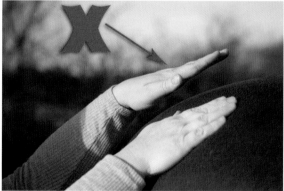

recipient! The sound that your hands make when they come into contact with the skin should be a hollow sound, rather than something that sounds like clapping or slapping.

Gently, gently – comfort is key

You can use cupping as firmly or as softly as you like. However, just to convince yourself that even a very soft cupping technique will have an effect, try using it as softly as you can on yourself or your partner, and decide whether you feel anything. Massage does not have to be high-pressure or forceful to be effective.

With any of these techniques, there is a tendency to believe that you have to press hard in order for the technique to be effective. The body is very clever, however, and even a light touch will be transferred through the layers of soft tissue and can have an effect deep within the body. It is more important to work slowly, to have the patience to massage for as long as necessary, and to stay focused with the intent to provide comfort, than it is to press hard.

Trust that it will become easier

Anything worth learning will take time to learn and perfect. Learning and practising these techniques and then massaging your horse will not feel any more natural to begin with than when you first learned to do rising trot or to drive a car! Take the time to practise, and read this chapter as many times as you need to until the techniques become clear. I've tried my best to explain in words and pictures something that is most easily demonstrated and corrected in person. However, in this way I can reach more horse owners and allow more horses to benefit from regular massage, which is something I am passionately committed to doing. You must trust that what initially seems complicated and awkward will gradually become second nature if you take the time to practise. Believe me, and the hundreds of others who have successfully learned these techniques and this routine before you and are now regularly massaging their own horses. The skill that you are learning is a skill for life, and it's worth taking the time to get it right.

2. Equine Anatomy

In this chapter you will:

- Learn about the seven key muscles (counting the pectoral group as one) that you will work on in the massage routine.

- Find out what these muscles do for your horse.

- See illustrations showing the relationship of the muscles to the skeleton.

- Learn how to chalk these muscles onto your own horse.

- Gain knowledge of how you can begin to relate performance problems to anatomy.

Understanding key muscle functions

In this chapter I give an overview of the whole body of the horse through selecting seven key muscles that cover a large proportion of the horse. Please don't get hung up on remembering the names of the muscles – think of them as labels necessary for me to be able to describe them to you. I've chosen muscles that I find are sore or tight in many of the horses that I treat.

I am going to explain what each of these key muscles does, discuss common causes of problems with each muscle, and describe how to chalk

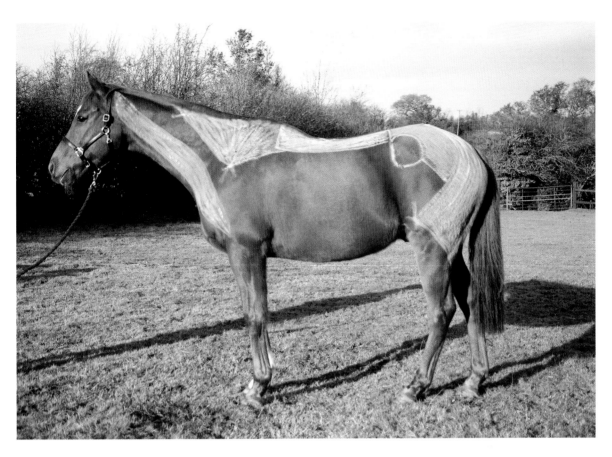

the muscles onto your horse. You will also find an illustration showing where each muscle is in relation to the skeleton of the horse. Alongside this illustration you will see accurate information regarding the action of the muscle (what it does), its origin (where it starts from) and its insertion (where it goes to). Some of this information is over and above what you need to know in order to be able to apply an effective and beneficial massage to your horse, but many of my students have been interested in this level of detail, and I've therefore included it for you.

Certainly, knowledge of the action of the muscle will enable you to understand better why it is important to massage that area. To determine what action the muscle has, we think about where it is attached at either end. Imagine the muscle like a piece of elastic that is held in mid-range, and so has the ability to either shorten or lengthen. If the elastic is shortened (i.e. the muscle contracts), the ends will move closer together. When the ends move apart, the elastic is lengthened (i.e. the

This chapter discusses seven key muscles in your horse.

muscle stretches). A muscle that is painful can act like elastic that is permanently shortened, and so can restrict movement. This has a knock-on effect throughout your horse's body.

Having a basic understanding of anatomy is not essential, but it's very useful. Knowing which bones the muscle attaches to gives you a good idea of what that muscle does. Knowing the action the muscle does gives you a good idea of what problems might be caused if that particular muscle is not working properly. You can then begin to relate performance problems in your horse to his underlying anatomy, and therefore address them with massage therapy. It's that simple (almost!). With this in mind I discuss the muscles, and in particular their actions, in an 'easy to follow' way, making learning anatomy interesting as well as educational. Your increased understanding will give you more confidence when you are working with your horse, and enhance your awareness of how, where and why you are applying your massage techniques.

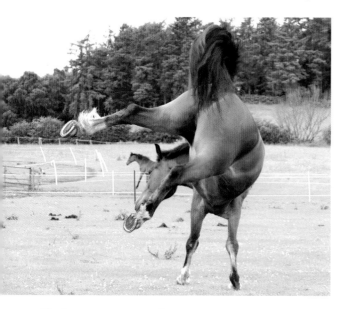

Having an awareness of potential problems means that you can begin to relate performance problems in your horse to the underlying anatomy, and address them with massage therapy.

Finding and chalking key muscles

I strongly encourage you to have a go at chalking the muscles onto your horse, as seen in the illustrations in this chapter. This is not only fun (and often satisfyingly messy!), but it really helps you to think about what lies beneath your horse's skin, and how you can influence him in a beneficial way. You cannot draw the muscles entirely accurately, but you can get close enough to deepen your understanding. Even just finding the landmarks to enable you to draw them will develop your awareness of your horse's anatomy. I explain in each section of this chapter how you can find the muscle and how you can draw it onto your horse. If you go wrong it doesn't matter; simply brush the dry chalk off and start again! The chalk I use is called 'giant chalk', 'playground chalk', or 'sidewalk chalk'. You can get your own from many places including Amazon or Hobbycraft.

To draw on your own horse, you need to immerse the chalk in water for a few minutes, and then use it while it is still wet. The chalk will only work when it is wet, and so you will have to wet it again if it starts to dry. Often when you first apply the wet chalk you can't see it straight away, but if you wait a few moments your lines will usually become clear as the chalk dries. To remove the chalk, simply brush your horse when the chalk is dry – it's that easy! *Warning: some coloured chalks on some horses may mark for a longer period – even up to a few days – in particular on grey horses, so please bear this in mind if you are planning on taking your horse out anywhere soon after drawing on him!*

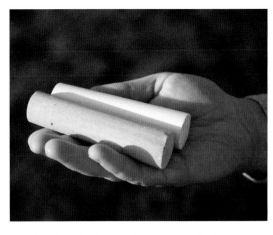

I explain in this chapter how you can find each muscle and draw it onto your horse.

The neck

Brachiocephalic muscle

Consists of *cleidocephalicus* muscle and *cleidobrachialis* muscle

Cleidocephalicus

Action: draws limb cranially, flexes head and rotates it laterally

Origin: clavicular intersection

Insertion: mastoid process of temporal bone

Cleidobrachialis

Action: draws limb cranially

Origin: clavicular intersection

Insertion: crest of humerus

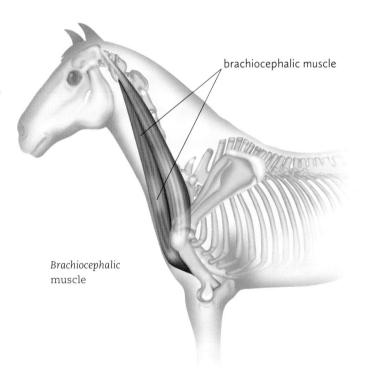

brachiocephalic muscle

Brachiocephalic muscle

It's all in the name

The *brachiocephalic* muscle is the neck muscle that you will concentrate on in your massage routine. The name sounds complicated, but in true anatomical fashion it simply describes where the muscle is in the body. *Brachio-* means 'arm' and '-*cephalic*' means 'head', so the *brachiocephalic* muscle goes from your horse's arm (the humerus, which is the bone between shoulder and elbow) to his head. As you can see from page 45, the muscle is anatomically described in two parts, the *cleidocephalicus* muscle and the *cleidobrachialis* muscle. '*Cleido-*' is a prefix meaning 'collarbone', so again these complicated-sounding names actually describe very simply where the muscle is situated – the *cleidocephalicus* muscle is the section of the *brachiocephalic* muscle from the collarbone region (I say 'region' because the horse does not actually have collarbones) to the head, and the *cleidobrachialis* muscle is the section from the collarbone region to the arm.

What the muscle does

If you think about the action that would occur if the *brachiocephalic* muscle was shortened (contracted), then your horse's head and 'arm' (i.e. his shoulder) would move towards each other. An important action of this muscle is moving his shoulder towards his poll, which brings the foreleg forwards. There is always a limit to how much a muscle can safely lengthen, and since the muscle is involved in moving the horse's foreleg forwards, it will also be involved in preventing his foreleg from going too far backwards when it reaches maximum stretch. Hence the *brachiocephalic* muscle is an important muscle when you are considering length of stride. If the muscle is damaged, tight or painful, then not only will it be less effective in moving your horse's foreleg forwards, it will also restrict the backwards movement, resulting in a shorter, choppier stride in front.

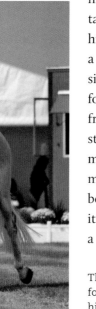

The *brachiocephalic* muscle brings the foreleg forwards out in front of your horse, and stops his foreleg from going too far underneath him.

Common causes of problems in the neck

Problems occur in the neck for many reasons; just some of them are listed here:

- A horse who is footsore or lame will show tension in the neck muscles near the shoulder.

- If your horse has had a heavy-handed rider or badly used 'gadgets' forcing his head into a certain position then the neck muscles will have suffered.

- Stiffness or soreness at the poll caused, for example, by a horse pulling back when he's tied up, will often work its way into the top of the neck muscles.

- A horse who jumps a lot, a driving horse or a horse who is working on hard ground will often be tight in his neck muscles.

Chalking on

To draw the *brachiocephalic* muscle on your horse, start by finding the bone at the top of your horse's neck (the atlas), just behind his ear. This is approximately the origin of the muscle. Then mark the point where your horse's shoulder joins his leg – this is effectively the insertion point of the muscle. The base of the muscle is easy to find – you can see the groove underneath your horse's neck (the jugular groove). To find the top of the muscle, place your fingers in the jugular groove and slide them across his neck towards his mane. About a third of the way between the jugular groove and the mane you will feel your fingers sink into his neck just a little. That's where you've come off the neck bones and sunk down into his neck muscle. Don't worry if you can't find it; just draw a line that divides the neck into one-third at the bottom and two-thirds at the top! Now that you've found the boundaries of the muscle, join the dots! Draw a line from the origin (poll) to insertion (shoulder) along the base of the muscle (the jugular groove), and from origin to insertion along the top of the muscle (one-third of the way up the neck). There's your *brachiocephalic* muscle!

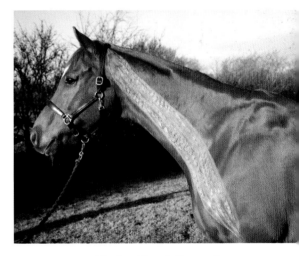

The *brachiocephalic* muscle goes from the poll to the shoulder.

The shoulder

Trapezius muscle

Action: draws limb cranially and abducts it; draws limb caudally and abducts it

Origin: nuchal ligament, and supraspinous ligament of C2 to T10

Insertion: cervical part – spine of scapula; thoracic part – proximal third of spine of scapula

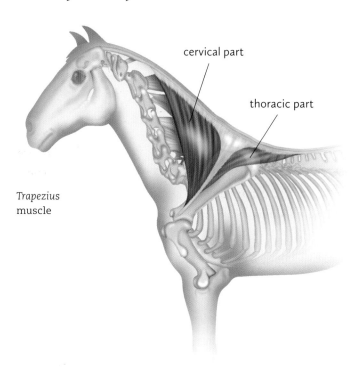

cervical part

thoracic part

Trapezius muscle

It's all in the name

The *trapezius* muscle is the shoulder muscle that you will concentrate on in your massage routine. It's easy to understand where the name came from for this one. If you look at the whole muscle from the top of the horse (i.e. the right side as well as the left side) then it's trapezius-shaped! You have the equivalent of the *trapezius* muscle in your own back; it acts to move your shoulder-blade and support your arm.

What the muscle does

The *trapezius* muscle attaches into the 'spine of scapula' (a ridge running the length of the shoulder-blade). This muscle has two portions, a cervical (neck) portion and a thoracic (chest) portion. The neck portion originates from a huge ligament in your horse's neck called the nuchal ligament (a broad elastic band of tissue connecting his neck bones to his withers), and from the lower neck bones. The chest portion originates from his withers. Both portions, when contracted, draw your horse's shoulder-blade upwards. If the neck portion is contracted, it will bring his shoulder-blade forwards, and if the chest portion is contracted it will bring his shoulder-blade backwards. Because of the action on the shoulder-blade, the *trapezius* muscle is involved in moving your horse's foreleg forwards and backwards. This means that, like the *brachiocephalic* muscle, the *trapezius* muscle will be involved in allowing and encouraging freedom of movement through his forehand.

Equally importantly, the action of the *trapezius* muscle is the opposite of that required for your horse to 'lift through his back', a phrase I'm sure many readers will be familiar with from their flatwork lessons. Soreness or dysfunction will cause contraction of the muscle and therefore restrict this movement, making it more difficult for your horse to work correctly.

Common causes of problems in the shoulder

Problems occur in the shoulder for many reasons; just some of them are listed here:

- Some of the thoracic portion of this shoulder muscle sits under the front of the saddle, and so poor saddle fit can have a detrimental effect on this muscle. The resulting soreness can mean that the horse hollows and shortens his stride in his ridden work to avoid the pain.

- A horse who is footsore, or lame in front for some other reason, may use the shoulder muscles to help try to take some of the weight off the sore leg, which could cause tension and soreness in the *trapezius* muscle.

- Jumping or working on hard ground can put extra strain through the shoulder muscles and related structures, which can lead to soreness.

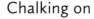

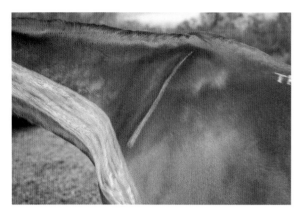

ABOVE To chalk the *trapezius* muscle onto your horse, first you need to find his 'spine of scapula'.

Chalking on

First you need to find your horse's 'spine of scapula'. Slide your hand down the upper half of your horse's neck until you get to the front of his shoulder-blade. Then look just a few centimetres further back and you will see a slight dip in the muscle structure. This dip runs diagonally down in roughly the same direction as the front of his shoulder-blade. If you press your fingers firmly into this dip and wriggle them forwards towards your horse's head and backwards towards his hock, you will feel a ridge of bone under your fingers. Follow this ridge up towards his withers and down towards his shoulder – this is the spine of scapula.

Now draw a cross about halfway down the spine of scapula (remember that these drawings are not totally accurate but are a rough guide for you to be able to massage effectively). Draw another cross just under your horse's mane halfway up his neck, and another on the top of his back under where his saddle would go. Now join the crosses, so that you have a triangular shape.

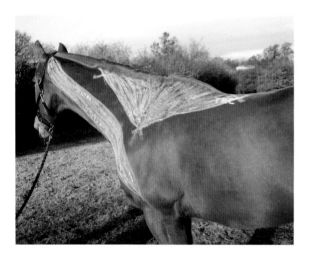

LEFT The *trapezius* muscle draws your horse's shoulder-blade upwards (and so tension in this muscle could restrict his 'lift through his back'), and is involved in the foreleg moving forwards and backwards.

The back

Longissimus dorsi muscle

Action: extends back and neck, stabilises vertebral column

Origin: wing of iliac bone, spinous processes of sacrum and lumbar and thoracic vertebrae

Insertion: transverse processes C4 to C7, and tubercles of ribs

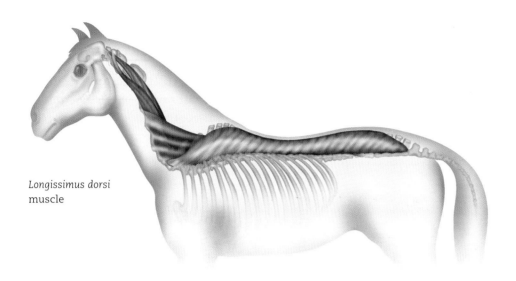

Longissimus dorsi muscle

It's all in the name

The *longissimus dorsi* muscle is the back muscle that you will concentrate on in your massage routine. '*Dorsi*' means back, and '*longissimus*' means 'long', so the *longissimus dorsi* muscle is quite literally the long back muscle. You have the equivalent muscle running down your back; it's a good muscle to work on if you practise your massage techniques on a partner.

What the muscle does

The *longissimus dorsi* muscle originates from the bones of your horse's pelvis and back, and attaches downwards, forwards and outwards from those bones onto the tops of his ribs at the rib angles, and to his neck bones at the base of his neck. Effectively this muscle runs all the way along his back and into his neck. Your horse's back naturally has a slight hollow, and if you think about the ends of his back being pulled together, contraction of the *longissimus dorsi* muscle will cause his back to hollow further. This is the opposite of what we look for from our horses in correct ridden work, when we ask them to 'work through their back'. Pain triggers contraction of a muscle, and therefore if pressure to the back

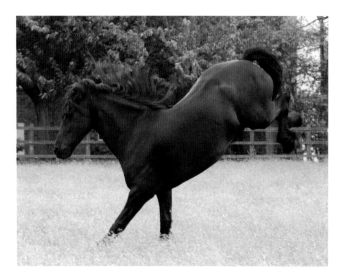

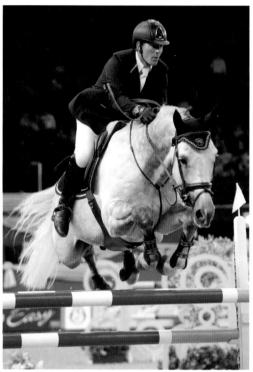

ABOVE Your horse's back naturally has a slight hollow, and contraction of the *longissimus dorsi* muscle will cause his back to hollow further.

RIGHT Your horse will only be able to round correctly and effortlessly through his back if it is not painful.

muscle is painful it will automatically contract and hollow your horse's back when you are sitting on him. This means that he will be unable to work as correctly as he is able to, even if he wants to.

Common causes of problems in the back

Problems occur in the back for many reasons; just some of them are listed here:

- A poorly fitting or poorly positioned saddle will put uneven pressure or too much pressure on the back muscle, causing pain and possibly loss of muscle tissue. You can imagine what this might feel like when you think of wearing a pair of shoes that are too small or don't fit.

- It is well established that lameness can lead to back pain, even if the lameness is so slight that it can't be seen or felt. This could be lameness in a fore or hind leg: the horse compensating for the problem by over-using his back muscles, or using them incorrectly, may cause the pain.

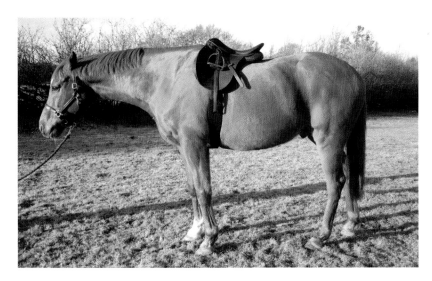

A poorly fitting or poorly positioned saddle will put uneven pressure or too much pressure on the *longissimus dorsi* muscle, causing pain and possibly loss of muscle tissue.

- Skeletal problems such as kissing spines (when the dorsal spinous processes are touching) can lead to back pain, including pain in the back muscles.

- A rider who is unbalanced will put uneven pressure through the horse's back, which could lead to pain in the back muscles.

Chalking on

You cannot get deep inside your horse to draw this muscle accurately, but you can draw an estimation of where it lies, for the purpose of massaging. You will, of course, then also benefit the other back muscles in the area, and any other connective tissue.

First run your hand over the upper part of your horse's shoulder-blade, and feel your hand move from hard cartilage and bone underneath his skin to soft tissue at the back of his shoulder-blade (many horses have a dip here, in the 'withers pocket', making the back of the shoulder-blade easy to see). Draw a vertical line downwards from his withers that runs level with the back of his shoulder-blade at this point. Next, draw a vertical line from the point where your horse's coat starts to change direction (just in front of his quarters) straight upwards to the top of his spine. Draw a horizontal line near the top of your horse's back, parallel to his spine but

BELOW To chalk the *longissimus dorsi* muscle onto your horse, first draw a vertical line downwards from his withers that runs down the back of his shoulder-blade at this point. Next, draw a vertical line from the point where his coat starts to change direction (near his point of hip) straight upwards to the top of his spine. Then draw a horizontal line parallel to his spine, and a horizontal line at the level of his rib angles.

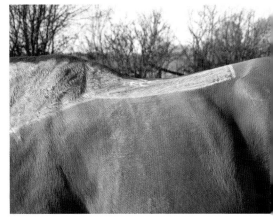

not quite as far up as the bony prominences – you should avoid massaging over bony areas, as it can be uncomfortable.

Find the top of your horse's ribcage (the rib angles) by pressing your fingers firmly into the middle of his ribcage at almost 90 degrees (do this carefully if your horse is ticklish). Slide your fingers upwards towards his back, until you feel them 'fall off' the ribcage into soft muscle. Be confident, and keep going until you find that soft muscle – many people stop too early. Draw a horizontal line at this level to join your line behind his shoulder-blade to your line where his coat changes direction. You now have a rectangle on your horse's back that denotes where you will massage to affect the back muscles.

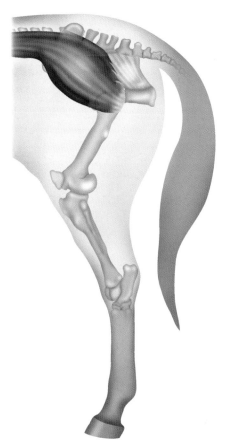

Gluteus medius muscle

The quarters

We will concentrate on three key muscles in the area of the quarters.

Gluteus medius muscle

Action: extends hip and rotates limb inward

Origin: lumbar part of *longissimus dorsi* muscle, gluteal surface of ilium, sacrum, sacroiliac ligament, broad sacrotuberous ligament

Insertion: greater trochanter

Biceps femoris muscle

Action: cranial part – extends hip and stifle joints, abducts limb; caudal part – flexes stifle and abducts limb, extends tarsal joint together with Achilles tendon

Origin: vertebral part – spinous and transverse processes of S3 to S5, broad sacrotuberous ligament, caudal fascia; pelvic part – ischial tuberosity

Insertion: patella, intermediate and lateral patellar ligaments; cranial border of tibia, crural fascia, common calcaneal tendon, and tuberosity of calcaneus

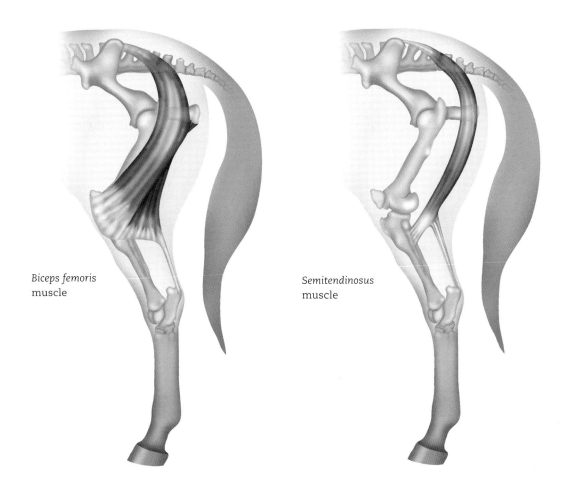

Biceps femoris
muscle

Semitendinosus
muscle

Semitendinosus muscle

Action: during weight bearing, extends hip, stifle and tarsal joints; when limb is not burdened, flexes stifle joint, draws limb backwards and rotates it inward

Origin: vertebral part – last sacral vertebra, transverse processes of S1 and S2, caudal fascia, broad sacrotuberous ligament; pelvic part – ventral part of ischial tuberosity

Insertion: cranial border of tibia, crural fascia, with tarsal ligament to tuberosity of calcaneus

It's all in the name

'*Gluteus*' comes from the Greek *gloutos* meaning 'buttock'. '*Medius*' means 'middle', so the *gluteus medius* muscle is the middle buttock muscle. There are two other gluteal muscles in the horse – *superficialis* (superficial) and *profundus* (deep). The labelling in the human is slightly different – you have a *gluteus maximus* muscle (biggest), a *gluteus medius* muscle, and a *gluteus minimus* muscle (smallest).

'*Bi-*' means 'two' and '*-ceps*' means 'head', so the *biceps* muscle has two 'heads' (two origins). '*Femoris*' means that it is related to the femur (thigh bone), so the *biceps femoris* muscle is a muscle with two origins that attaches into the thigh bone. You have the equivalent muscle in the back of your thigh.

'*Semi-*' means 'half' and '*-tendinosus*' is related to tendon, so it makes sense that the *semitendinosus* muscle has an exceptionally long tendon. Again you have the equivalent muscle in the back of your thigh.

What these muscles do

The *gluteus medius* muscle is one of your horse's three gluteal muscles. The gluteal muscles as a group are crucial to the power of the horse. The *biceps femoris* muscle and the *semitendinosus* muscle are two of his three 'hamstring' muscles (the third being the *semimembranosus* muscle). You will no doubt be familiar with the phrase 'hamstring muscle' relating to the muscles that run down the back of your thigh, since a 'torn hamstring' is a common football injury. The *gluteus medius* muscle and the hamstring muscles are involved in moving your horse's hind leg backwards (extending the hip). The other gluteal muscles have different actions.

This means that, when your horse steps forwards and puts his weight through one hind leg, the *gluteus medius* muscle, the *biceps femoris* muscle

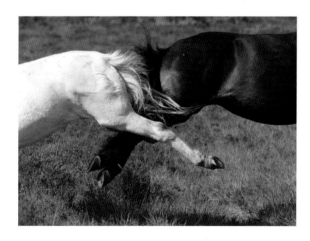

The *gluteus medius* muscle and the hamstring muscles are involved in moving the hind leg backwards.

and the *semitendinosus* muscle act to bring that leg backwards. The result of this is that your horse's body moves forwards over the leg to enable him to step forwards onto the other leg. In the horse, these muscles are involved in galloping, in the take-off for jumping, and in bucking or kick-ing (not that these are behaviours that you are likely to encourage in his ridden work!). For your horse to be able to work efficiently his gluteal muscles and his hamstring muscles must be free from pain or tension.

Thinking about the action of these muscles being one of bringing your horse's hind leg backwards, you will see that they also act as a 'brake' for his hind leg going forwards, resisting too much forward movement to ensure that the leg doesn't move further than its maximum stretch. Therefore, any restriction to his gluteal muscles and his hamstring muscles, such as that caused by soreness or stiffness, will mean that his hind leg isn't able to come as far forwards under him as it would do otherwise. Clearly this will have an effect on his ability to 'overtrack', on stride length, and on the ability of your horse to engage through his hindquarters.

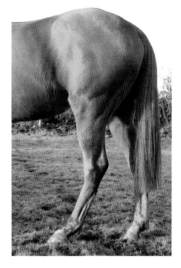

ABOVE Restriction to the hamstrings, such as that caused by soreness or stiffness, will mean that the hind leg isn't able to come as far forwards under your horse. Clearly this will have an effect on his ability to 'overtrack', and his ability to engage through his hindquarters.

Common causes of problems in the quarters

Problems occur in the quarters for many reasons; just some of them are listed here:

- Hind limb lameness will result in pain in the muscles of the quarters as they have to work harder to try to avoid putting too much weight through that leg.

- Long-term pain in the hind limb will result in the horse using his hind end unevenly, and the muscles in the quarters will adjust to compensate for this. The likely result is pain and/or stiffness.

- Overwork will lead to soreness and tightness in the muscles of the quarters, and introducing new work may also do this, in just the same way that your muscles will ache if you spend longer in the gym than you are used to. This is particularly the case in horses who are jumping, galloping, or performing high-level dressage movements.

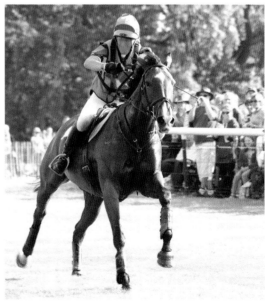

RIGHT Overwork, or introducing new work, could lead to soreness and tightness in the hamstrings.

- A horse who is stiff or functioning poorly elsewhere in his body will often have soreness through the muscles in his quarters, through compensatory movements.

Chalking on

Start with your horse's *semitendinosus* muscle. Draw a line from where his tail joins his body, directly down the back of his quarters to a point level with his stifle (be sure to keep yourself safe, if your horse is sore or sensitive here then he might kick out). Then find the 'racing line' or 'poverty line' (which marks the junction between the *semitendinosus* muscle and *biceps femoris* muscle) and draw a line there, that starts and finishes in the same place as your first line. This is the *semitendinosus* muscle, for the purposes of your massage routine.

Next, draw his *biceps femoris* muscle. Draw a cross halfway along your horse's quarters, on his spine. Draw another cross close to his stifle (be careful, lots of horses are ticklish here). Now join the dots! The cross on his spine is joined to the cross on the stifle by a curve; on his off side (right side), it will be like a big 'C'; on his near side (left side) it will be like a back to front 'C'. Join the cross on his stifle to the bottom of the

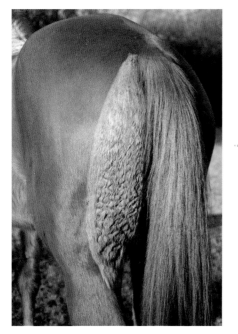

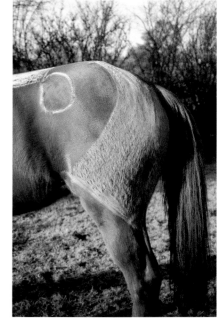

LEFT The *semintendinosus* muscle runs down the back of your horse's hind leg from near the top of his tail.

RIGHT The *biceps femoris* muscle is a powerful hamstring muscle that runs from near the top of your horse's tail towards his stifle.

semitendinosus muscle with a straight line. You will see that the *biceps femoris* muscle is a big, powerful muscle in the horse!

Find your horse's point of hip (it's anatomically known as the tuber coxae) – the bony area near the top of where his coat changes direction on his flanks. Have a feel of the section of his pelvic bone that lies quite close under the skin in this area, and draw a big circle (which will look more like a kidney shape if you can feel the bone clearly) around that area. As mentioned earlier, you should avoid massaging over bone as this could be uncomfortable for your horse.

Next, draw a line from the back of that circle, diagonally downwards to meet the front of your horse's *biceps femoris* muscle. Everything on his quarters above that diagonal line is what you're going to think of as his *gluteus medius* muscle (remember that you can't be entirely accurate in your chalking, but it's close enough for the purposes of your massage routine).

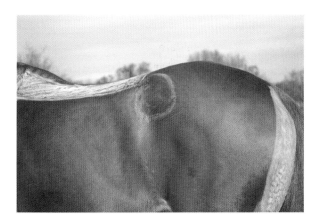

Draw a line around the point of hip. You want to avoid massaging over this bony area as it could be uncomfortable for your horse.

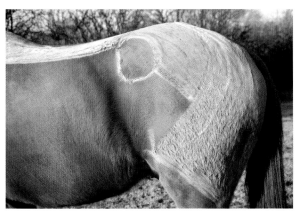

The *gluteus medius* muscle is a powerful muscle running from your horse's pelvis to his low back.

The chest

We will concentrate on three key muscles in the chest area. While their key individual characteristics are outlined below, for the general purposes of this book we are going to consider them as a group.

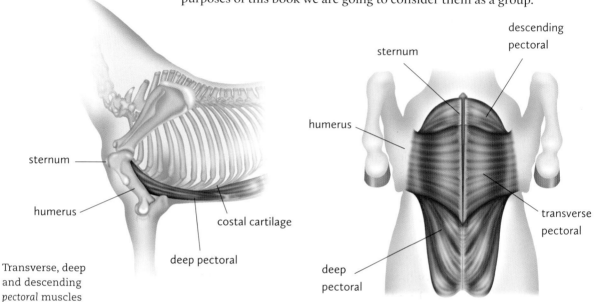

Transverse, deep and descending *pectoral* muscles

The superficial pectoral muscles

Transverse superficial *pectoral* muscle and cranial superficial *pectoral* muscle

Action: attach limb to trunk, adduct limb

Origin: transverse – costal cartilages 1 to 6, sternum; cranial – manubrium of sternum

Insertion: transverse – antebrachial fascia; cranial – crest of humerus, antebrachial fascia

Deep *pectoral* muscle

Action: supports trunk, adducts limb and draws it caudally, stabilises shoulder joint

Origin: sternum, costal cartilages 4 to 9, and yellow abdominal tunic

Insertion: greater and lesser tubercles of humerus, antebrachial fascia

It's all in the name

The name 'pectoral' comes from the Latin pectus meaning 'heart' or 'breast'. The pectoral muscles are attached to the breast bone of the horse. You have pectoral muscles that run from your breast bone to your arm; you can often find them as a tender spot if you prod either side of your breast bone just underneath your collarbone.

What these muscles do

Your horse doesn't have a collarbone, so he doesn't have the same bony attachment of limb to spine as you do as a human. In your horse it is purely soft tissue (which includes tendons, ligaments and fascia as well as muscle) that keeps his forelimbs close to his neck, back and ribcage. The pectoral muscles are one group of muscles that do this. They also support the trunk of your horse from underneath. For him to be able to 'lift through his back', his pectoral muscles have got to contract to lift his spine and ribcage (in conjunction with contraction and relaxation of a variety of other muscles). For him to move freely through his forehand, his pectoral muscles have to be relaxed and supple enough to allow that movement. If you clamp your upper arm against your sides and then try

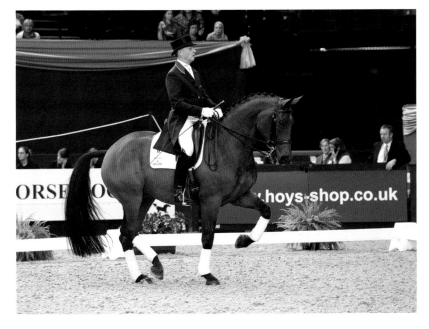

The pectoral muscles support the trunk of your horse from underneath. For your horse to be able to 'lift through his back', these muscles have got to contract to lift his spine and ribcage.

moving your arms, you will have an idea of how restricted your horse's movement might be if his *pectoral* muscles are tight.

Common causes of problems in the chest

Problems occur in the chest for many reasons; just some of them are listed here:

- Poorly fitting saddles will put strain through the chest muscles as they are unable to support the trunk effectively during your ridden work, and the result may be soreness.

- The wrong kind of girth for your horse may cause bruising through the chest muscles (and other muscles).

- Restricted side flexion of the neck (either through your ridden work, or through an inherent stiffness in your horse) may lead to irritation of the nerves that supply the chest muscles, and the result could be apparent soreness and sensitivity (often thought of as 'ticklishness').

- Hard ground or lameness, where the horse naturally restricts his length of stride, can lead to tightness through the chest muscles.

Chalking on

I recommend that you look and feel for the *pectoral* muscles rather than chalking them on in case your horse, like many others, is sore in this area.

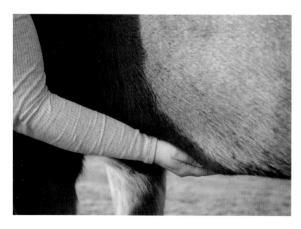

I don't recommend that you chalk the chest muscles onto your horse, partly because it would be very difficult to see the results, and partly because so many horses are sore through this area that I don't want to risk irritating them. Instead, I recommend that you look and feel for these muscles. They are easy to see from the front: you might have heard them being called 'horse boobs'! Often you can see, and can certainly feel, a bulge either side of your horse's breast bone. If you follow the muscle on one side down between his forelegs and continue on through the girth area and along the midline towards the back of the horse, you will feel that you 'fall off' the muscle about a third of the way along his tummy. If you're struggling to find the place that you 'fall off', move your hand back to your horse's elbow and stroke

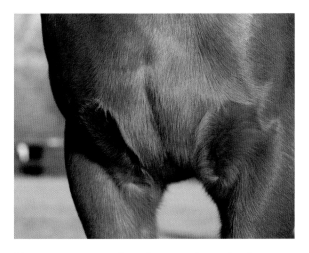

It's easy to spot your horse's pectoral muscles from in front; they may have previously been referred to as his 'horse boobs'.

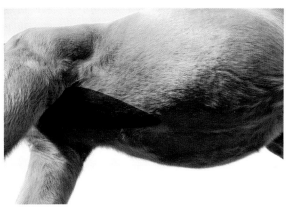

If you follow the muscle on one side down between your horse's forelegs and continue on through his girth area and along his midline towards the rear of the horse, you will feel that you 'fall off' the muscle about a third of the way along his tummy.

back towards his stifle, keeping about a hand's width from his midline – sometimes the border of the muscle is easier to feel here. People are often surprised just how big the chest muscles are – they are powerful and important muscles and yet I often find that soreness in this area is just dismissed as 'girthiness' or 'ticklishness'.

3. Massaging Your Horse

In this chapter you will:

- Learn how to put into practise on your horse the techniques you discovered in the first chapter.

- Find out how to apply these techniques to the neck, shoulders, back, quarters and chest of your horse.

- Develop a massage routine that you can use with your own horse, and with practice become confident in using this routine on a regular basis.

- At the end of the book is a 'prompt section', a shorthand version of the routine that you can use when you are working with your horse.

Safety first

When you are massaging your horse, safety is of the utmost importance. Massage should be an enjoyable and relaxing way of spending time with your horse, so it is worth taking some simple precautions to ensure this is the case.

Wearing sensible clothing and footwear will mean that you are more relaxed and comfortable around your horse as well as being safer. You should remove rings, watches and bracelets for the comfort of yourself and of your horse.

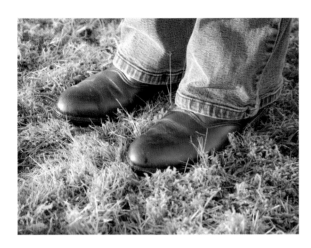

Wearing sensible clothing and footwear, such as steel toe-capped boots, will mean that you are more comfortable around your horse as well as being safer.

Take care of your own body. Think about your posture, the direction that your feet and hips are pointing, the way you are holding your wrists and the way that you are using your fingers. Try different positions until you find ones that are comfortable for you.

Where you massage your horse can make a big difference to his relaxation and comfort levels. This could be in his stable, in the yard, or in his field, wherever you and he feel relaxed and happy. It will be easier, though, if he is dry and relatively clean. Make sure that the surrounding area is safe and relatively free from distractions. Take a good look all around you before you begin.

If you decide to stand on a mounting block to be able to reach your horse more easily, make sure that the block is safe and secure, and that you can move it to wherever your horse is most comfortable. The block should be strong and solid in case your horse steps towards or onto it by mistake.

For most horses, the neck or the shoulder is a good place to begin – they are happy with you working in this area and are used to being stroked and patted there. However, if your horse is uncomfortable with you working there for whatever reason, then try starting somewhere that he is comfortable with. If he still seems uncomfortable and reactive to your touch, consider calling a professional such as your vet or physiotherapist to assess him further.

It is advisable to have a handler holding your horse for the first couple of massage sessions, until you know how he will react to your touch and you are more able to concentrate on him. Communication with the

A handler should stand on the same side of the horse as you are working, so that if your horse needs to move, they can direct his head towards them and therefore his quarters away from you.

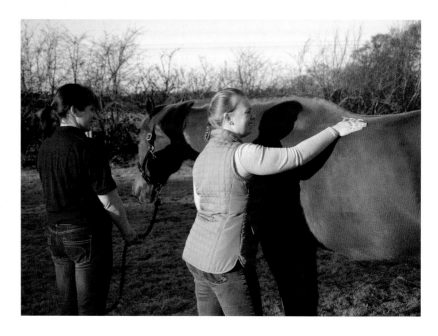

handler, as well as with your horse, is essential. This means explaining to your handler what you are going to do and when you are going to do it, and not making any surprise moves. Your handler should retain a loose hold on the rope so that your horse doesn't feel that he needs to pull or push into the pressure of the rope. They should stand on the same side of the horse as you are working, so that if your horse needs to move, they can direct his head towards them and therefore his quarters away from you.

Communication with your horse means, amongst everything else, keeping a close eye on your horse's reactions and responding accordingly. Keeping at least one hand on your horse at all times will mean that you don't surprise him and are therefore less likely to trigger an instinctive 'fight or flight' reaction. Remember that, if you find a sore spot, your horse may let you know in a number of ways, which can include biting, kicking, and moving sharply. Be prepared; observe your horse at all times for signs of how he is feeling about his massage, and allow him to communicate with you in a safe way.

Observe your horse at all times for signs of how he is feeling about his massage, and allow him to communicate with you in a safe way.

Contraindications and precautions

A contraindication is something that means you should definitely *not* massage your horse. A precaution is something that means you should make an educated decision, supported by your vet, as to whether or not you should massage him, or is something that you should be aware of whilst you are massaging.

Contraindications

Never massage your horse without the consent of your vet if:

- He has a problem that has not been properly diagnosed. There is the potential that you could make the problem worse.

- You see abnormal swelling, or feel abnormal temperature changes (usually heat). There is the potential you could cause further damage.

- He has an elevated pulse, respiration rate, or temperature. A horse with any of these signs needs veterinary attention.

- Your horse has azoturia (also known traditionally as 'tied-up', 'Monday morning disease' and 'setfast', and now termed 'exertional rhabdomyolysis'). Massage could worsen the problem.

- He is suffering from an infection. Massage could cause the infection to spread more quickly.

- He has an infectious skin condition. Massage could contribute to the spread of the infection, both throughout your horse and to yourself.

- There is recent injury. In this case you should seek veterinary advice.

Precautions

Be cautious working with your horse when:

- He has an open wound. You should avoid working close to the wound as this could be painful for him and could lead to infection.

- He is lame. I recommend that you discuss with your vet if you are in any way unsure whether or not massage is appropriate.

- Any cancerous tumours or cysts are present. There may be the potential that massage could spread them; again discuss your horse's individual case with your vet.

The massage routine

It cannot be stressed enough how important it is to listen to your horse. As your technique improves, you will be better able to read your horse's reactions and feel the areas where he would like more pressure and the areas where he would like you to ease off. To begin with, work softly and slowly. Keep at least one hand on your horse at all times, to maintain the flow of energy.

You can begin your massage on the left (near) or the right (off) side of your horse. I am going to describe the routine with you beginning on his left side.

Beginning

1. To begin with, stroke your horse gently and slowly over his whole body, working from the front of his body towards the back. Use this time to put the stresses of daily life aside, and to find the calm place in your mind where you can enjoy time with your horse. I often talk

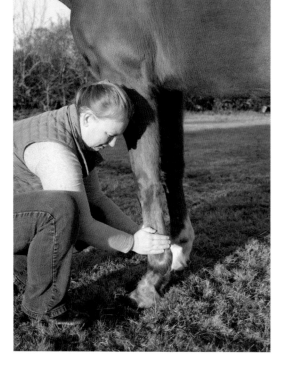

about leaving all your worries at the stable door or the field gate. You are, of course, welcome to pick them up again on the way out of the stable or field once you have finished massaging your horse!

Use this initial time to assess your horse's general health and wellbeing. Can you feel any lumps, bumps, or swellings, or anywhere that is warmer or colder than expected? Does he feel particularly tight anywhere, or over-reactive, sore, or even ticklish? Compare the left side of your horse to his right side. Are there any minor cuts that you weren't aware of (or even more major wounds)? Feel down his legs as well as along his body, and include his head, his ears and his poll, underneath his tail, in between his forelegs and in between his hind legs if it's safe to do so. Repeat this exercise on each side of your horse.

To begin with, assess your horse's overall health and wellbeing. Feel down his legs as well as over his body.

The neck

2. Start your massage with effleurage on your horse's neck.

- Apply effleurage from the point of your horse's shoulder towards his poll, applying slow, gentle pressure.

- At or near the poll, release any pressure, keeping your hand in contact with your horse, and slide your hand back towards his point of shoulder.

- Take about four seconds to apply effleurage from shoulder to poll, and about four seconds to slide from poll back to shoulder.

- Use the hand nearer your horse's head to perform the massage move, and rest the other hand against his shoulder or ribcage.

- Be aware of your posture. Stand comfortably with your feet slightly apart and your knees soft.

- Repeat this move three times.

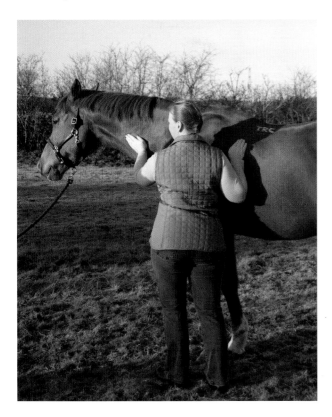

LEFT Start your massage with effleurage on your horse's neck. Apply effleurage from the point of your horse's shoulder towards his poll. Use the hand nearer your horse's head to perform the massage move, and rest the other hand against his shoulder or ribcage.

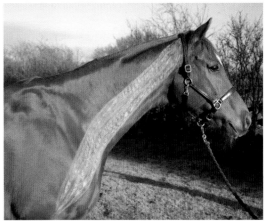

ABOVE The *brachiocephalicus* muscle runs from the shoulder to the poll.

3. Next, use compression to soften your horse's neck muscle. The compression move is done from your horse's poll towards his shoulder.

- Begin where you finished the effleurage motion, at the point of shoulder. It's important in this massage routine that one technique moves smoothly into another without any loss of contact between you and your horse.

- Slide your hand lightly towards your horse's poll, and then use compressions as you move back down towards his shoulder.

- Slide the skin away from you towards his ears in each compression move.

- Use between four and ten compressions along the length of the neck, depending on how big your horse is and how much time you have available. More compressions will lead to greater relaxation of the muscle, but will take more time.

- Think of the compression as a four-second move – take one second to gently squash into the muscle, one second to slide the skin up towards your horse's poll, one second to release the pressure, and one second to slide your hand to the next spot.

- Repeat this move three times.

Next, use compression to soften your horse's neck muscle. Slide your hand lightly towards your horse's poll, and then use compressions as you move back down towards your horse's shoulder. Think of the compression as a four-second move – take one second to press gently into the muscle, one second to slide the skin up towards your horse's poll, one second to release the pressure, and one second to slide your hand to the next spot.

4 sec

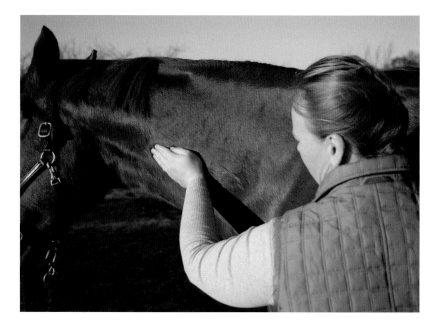

4. Apply effleurage three times over the neck muscle as in step two.

5. Repeat steps two to four on the right side of your horse.

The shoulder

6. Moving on to the shoulder, we again use effleurage, then compression, and finish by repeating the effleurage. To get started with effleurage, we need to plan the direction of our techniques, since this muscle is wider than the *brachiocephalicus* muscle.

   - Draw in your mind (or with chalk) some lines on the *trapezius* muscle. The first and fifth lines are the 'V' that you drew when you chalked the outline of the muscle. It starts from halfway down your horse's spine of scapula (shoulder-blade) to a point under his mane halfway up his neck, and to a point on his back under where his saddle would go. The third line goes from the starting point on the spine of scapula directly towards his withers. The second and fourth lines split each half of the muscle in half again, so that you have divided the *trapezius* muscle into four, like pizza slices!

   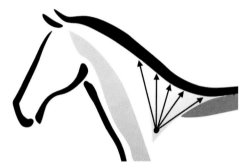

   The *trapezius* muscle connects the shoulder-blade to the trunk. Draw in your mind (or with chalk) some lines on this shoulder muscle.

   - Your effleurage moves on your horse's shoulder region always begin with both hands together at the point where the lines meet.

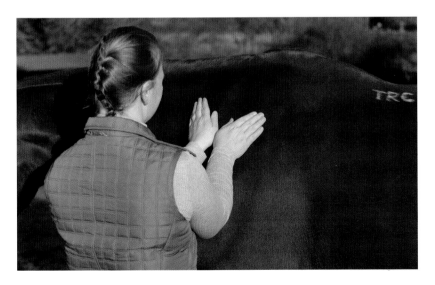

Your effleurage moves on the shoulder region always begin with both hands together at the point where the lines meet.

- First apply effleurage with both hands at the same time away from you along the outer lines (the first 'V' that you drew), so that the hand nearer your horse's head travels from his shoulder on to his neck, and the hand nearer your horse's tail travels from his shoulder on to his back. Then release the pressure and slide your hands back to the starting point.

- Next apply effleurage away from you along the second and fourth lines (the quarter and three-quarter lines) again using both hands at the same time, then release the pressure and slide back to the beginning.

- Finally, use both hands away from you along the line towards the withers, then release the pressure and slide back.

- In each case, take around four seconds to move from the starting point to the furthest point away, and then around four seconds to slide your hands back to the starting point.

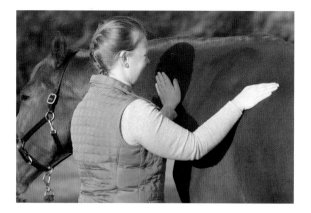

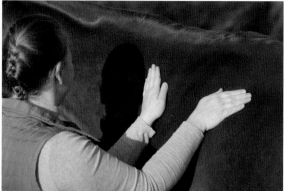

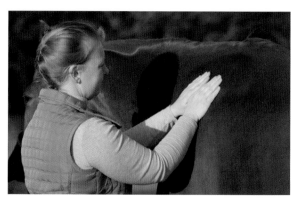

ABOVE LEFT First, apply effleurage with both hands along the outer lines.

ABOVE RIGHT Next, apply effleurage with both hands along the middle lines.

RIGHT Then apply effleurage with both hands along the inner line.

- Repeat this routine three times along each of the three lines. Your hands will finish over the point that is part-way down the shoulder-blade.

7. Next, use compression to address the shoulder region through the *trapezius* muscle. The compression move uses the same three lines that were used in the effleurage move.

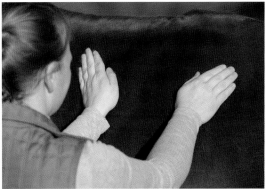

- Continuing smoothly on from finishing the effleurage move, you will start with your hands over the point on your horse's shoulder-blade.

- Slide both hands slowly to the far end of the outside lines of the trapezius muscle, so that one hand is under the horse's mane halfway up his neck, and the other hand is on his back in the saddle region.

- Move your hands gradually back towards your starting point on your horse's shoulder-blade, using between four and ten compressions along the way.

Next use compression to address the shoulder region through the *trapezius* muscle. Always slide the skin away from you during the 'glide' part of the compression move.

- Always slide the skin away from you during the 'glide' part of the compression move.

- Keep your hands in harmony with each other. Each compression should take around four seconds.

- Next, slide both hands out along the second and fourth lines, and compress back towards your starting point, again using between four and ten compressions.

- Then slide both hands together towards your horse's withers along your inner line, once more using between four and ten compressions as you return to the starting point that is halfway down the shoulder-blade.

- Repeat this routine three times along each of the three lines.

8. Apply effleurage over the *trapezius* muscle as in step six.

9. Repeat steps six to eight on the right side of your horse.

The back

10. To massage the back muscles (including the *longissimus dorsi* muscle), I again suggest using effleurage, then compression, and then effleurage. By now you will be getting comfortable with this pattern, and the techniques will be starting to feel familiar. As you become more confident, you will be able to concentrate less on what you are doing with your hands and more on what you are feeling. You will then start to be able to recognise when your horse's muscles are in good health and when they are in need of treatment. To begin with, use effleurage.

- Rest the hand nearer your horse's head on the side of his neck or shoulder; this hand is not involved in massaging his back. Slide your other hand to his back below his withers, just behind the shoulder-blade.

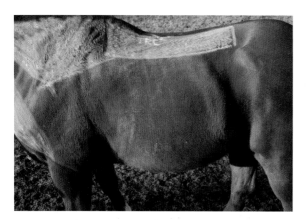

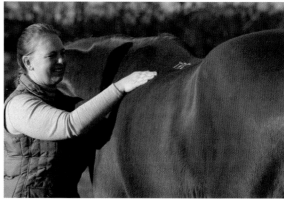

ABOVE LEFT The *longissimus dorsi* muscle is one of the long back muscles. To massage the back muscles, I suggest using effleurage, then compression, then effleurage again.

ABOVE RIGHT The starting point for both the effleurage and the compression moves along your horse's back is the junction where the top of the ribcage meets the back of the shoulder-blade.

- The starting point for both the effleurage and the compression moves along your horse's back is the junction where the top of his ribcage meets the back of his shoulder-blade. You drew this as the bottom front corner of the rectangle on your horse's back that represented the *longissimus dorsi* muscle.

- Similar to when working on the *trapezius* muscle, start by drawing three lines along your horse's back muscle to guide you in each move. Remembering the rectangle that you chalked on his back, the first line for your massage moves goes from the bottom front corner of that rectangle to the top back corner, on his back above where his coat changes direction.

- The second line goes from the bottom front corner to a spot halfway along the top line of the rectangle, which is halfway along your horse's back.

- The third line goes from the bottom front corner of the rectangle to the top front corner, at his withers.

- Apply effleurage along each of these lines, the first, then the second, then the third, applying pressure as your hand moves away from you, and releasing this pressure as you slide your hand back towards you.

- Take around four seconds to apply effleurage away from you along each line, and around four seconds to slide your hand back to the starting point each time.

- Repeat this three times along each of the three lines.

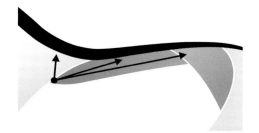

Similar to the *trapezius* muscle, you need to draw three lines along the *longissimus dorsi* muscle to guide each effleurage move.

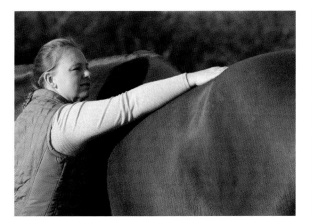

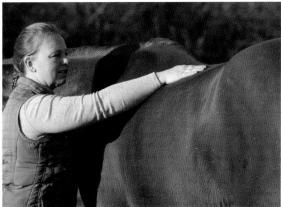

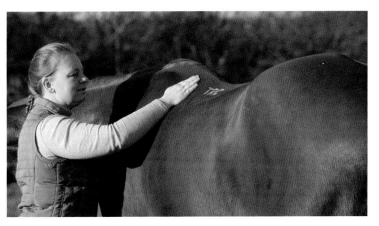

ABOVE LEFT Apply effleurage along the first line.

ABOVE RIGHT Then along the second line.

RIGHT Continue by applying effleurage along the third line.

11. Follow your effleurage with the compression technique along each of these lines.

    - Keep the hand nearer your horse's head resting softly against his neck or shoulder, and start your compression move from the point just behind his shoulder-blade where you started each of the effleurage moves.

    - Slide your hand to the end of the first line, on your horse's back above where his coat changes direction, then use the compression move as you return to your starting point.

    - Work in the same way along the second and the third lines, always sliding the skin away from you during the compression move.

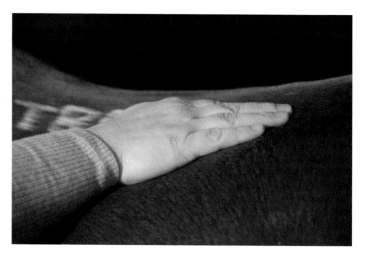

Follow the effleurage with the compression technique along each of these lines. Slide your hand to the end of the line, and then use the compression move as you return to your starting point. Always slide the skin away from you during the compression move.

    - Use between four and ten compression moves along each line; each compression should take around four seconds.

    - Repeat this three times along each of the three lines.

12. Apply effleurage over your horse's back muscles as in step ten.

13. Repeat steps ten to twelve on the right side of your horse.

The quarters

14. To massage your horse's quarters, we combine the *gluteus medius* muscle, the *biceps femoris* muscle and the *semitendinosus* muscle into one area. Here you will use effleurage again but then, instead of compression, I suggest kneading and cupping, followed once more by effleurage. That is not to say that you can't use compression on the quarters, or kneading and cupping elsewhere, only that I have chosen these techniques for this particular routine. We begin with effleurage.

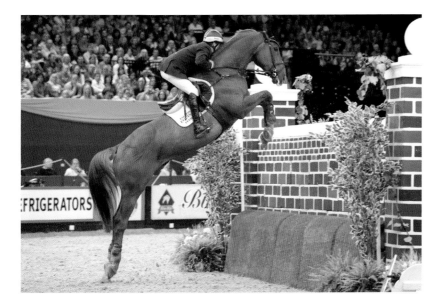

The quarters are where the power comes from.

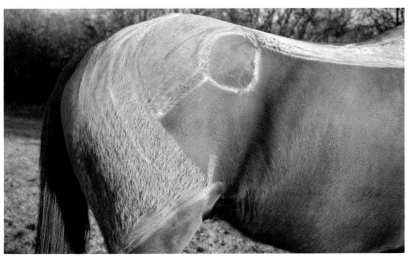

On the quarters I suggest using effleurage again, but then instead of compression, I recommend kneading and cupping, followed of course by effleurage.

- Keep at least one of your hands in contact with your horse as you change position to be able to massage his quarters. Ensure that you are standing in a safe position before you begin.

- For effleurage, we again start by dividing the area up with three lines. Each of the lines starts from the hip, so your first task is to find your horse's hip. To do this, find your horse's seat bone, which is the furthest point back on his body. It's generally (depending on the size of your horse) about a hand's width down from the top of the tail. Then slide your fingers, in a direction parallel to the ground, around his quarters towards the front, stopping about one-third of the way between his seat bone and the point where his coat changes direction at the front of his quarters. If you still have the quarter muscles chalked on, this will be roughly where the *biceps femoris* muscle meets the *semitendinosus* muscle. On some horses you can feel the top of the thigh bone under your fingers as a bony prominence under the skin; this indicates that you are close to his hip.

- With your horse's hip as your starting point, the first line goes to meet the point at which you finished massaging his back muscle, on his back above where his coat changes direction. Draw this on with chalk, or with your finger. The second line goes from his hip to a point on his spine halfway between the top of his tail and the point above where his coat changes direction. The third line goes from his hip to the top of his tail.

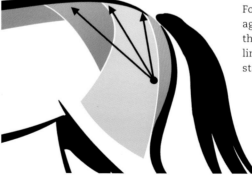

For the effleurage, we again need to divide the area up with three lines. Each of the lines starts from the hip.

- Rest the hand nearer your horse's head softly against his ribcage, and work with the hand nearer his tail.

- Apply effleurage on each of the three lines, applying pressure as you move away from his hip, and releasing the pressure to slide back to your starting point.

- Take around four seconds to move your hand away from his hip, and around four seconds to lightly slide your hand back again.

- Repeat this three times along each of the three lines.

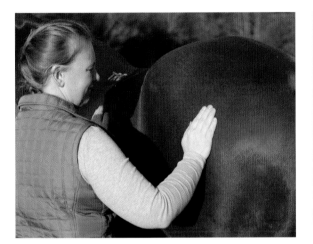
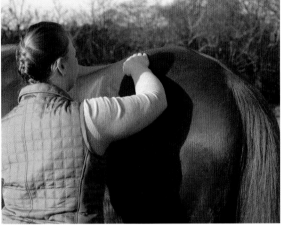
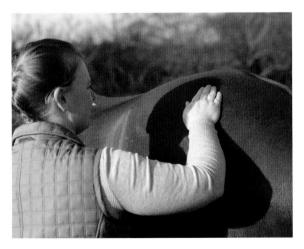
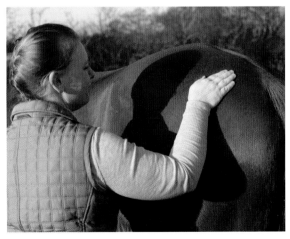

TOP LEFT With the hip as your starting point, rest the hand nearer your horse's head softly against your horse's ribcage, and work with the hand nearer your horse's tail.

TOP RIGHT, BELOW LEFT AND RIGHT Apply effleurage along each of the three lines, applying pressure as you move away from your horse's hip, and releasing the pressure to slide back to your starting point.

15. Follow your effleurage with kneading.

- Use the hand nearer your horse's tail to knead his quarters gently, and keep the hand nearer his head resting gently on his ribcage.

- There doesn't need to be a particular pattern to your kneading. You can choose to follow the three lines or you can choose to knead in a random fashion throughout your horse's quarters.

- Remember that you can only twist your horse's skin and muscles within the range that they're able to move. If your hand slides *over* his hair rather than *with* it, then you have moved further than his skin is able to stretch.

- Different areas of his quarters will feel very different from each other, depending on the structures underneath his skin. Work in a way that feels comfortable to both you and your horse.

- Take around four seconds for each kneading move. It takes time for the tension to release from his skin, muscles and other tissues.

BELOW LEFT Follow the effleurage with kneading. Use the hand nearer your horse's tail to knead his quarters gently, and keep the hand nearer his head resting gently on his ribcage.

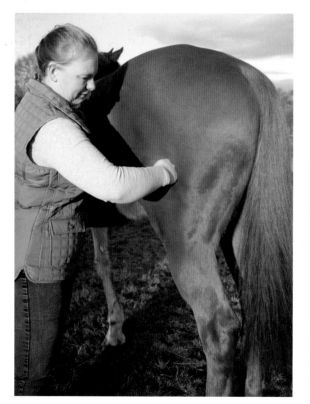

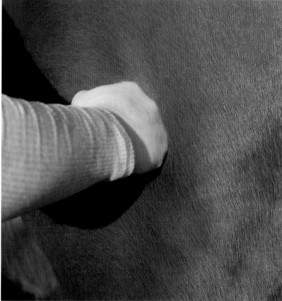

ABOVE Remember with kneading that you can only twist the skin and muscles within the range that they're able to move. If your hand slides over the hair, rather than with the hair, then you have moved further than the skin is able to.

- Avoid kneading over bony areas, as this might be uncomfortable for your horse.

- Knead over your horse's quarters for around one minute, or longer if you prefer.

16. After kneading, use gentle cupping over your horse's quarters.

    - As with the effleurage and the kneading, work across his *gluteus medius* muscle, his *biceps femoris* muscle and his *semitendinosus* muscle as one group.

    - Use both hands alternately for cupping.

    - Work gently in a steady rhythm, and look for your cupping technique to cause a slight 'wobble' through your horse's muscles around the area that you're working.

    - There is no set pattern to the cupping; work wherever is comfortable for you and your horse. Often this is along the top or down the back of his quarters.

    - Use the cupping technique for around thirty seconds, or longer if you prefer.

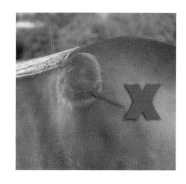

Avoid kneading over bony areas, as this might be uncomfortable for your horse.

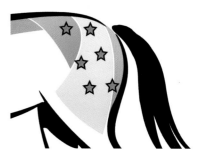

ABOVE After kneading, use gentle cupping over the quarters. There is no set pattern to the cupping; work wherever is comfortable for you and your horse.

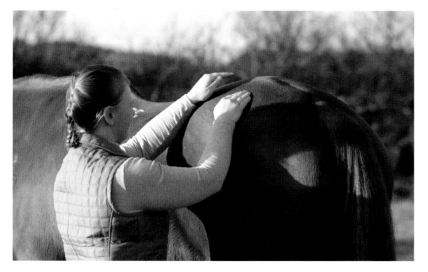

LEFT Use both hands for cupping. Work very gently in a steady rhythm, and look for your cupping technique to cause a slight 'wobble' through your horse's muscle around the area that you're working.

17. Apply effleurage your horse's quarters as in step 14.

18. Repeat steps 14 to 17 on the right side of your horse.

The chest

19. For the chest, effleurage is the only technique that I am recommending to begin with. For one thing, effleurage is incredibly effective. Also, so many horses are sore or hypersensitive in this area that it wouldn't be fair to use the other techniques until they were more comfortable. Once you are more confident massaging your horse you may wish to include a wider variety of techniques in this area.

- Keep one hand on your horse as you change position. Stand beside him facing his shoulder, with your feet apart and your knees bent, so that you can reach his chest and between his forelegs without having to bend your back.

- Start with the hand nearer your horse's head (we'll call that the left hand since I'm suggesting that you start on the left side of your horse) at the top of the pectoral muscle group, on his 'horse boob' on the side nearer you. Keep the other hand (your right hand) free, as you'll be using it in a moment.

- Slide your left hand down over the muscle and between your horse's forelegs, keeping to the side of the muscle that you started on.

- When your left hand is as far as you can reach between his forelegs, place your right hand on top of your left hand and use your right hand to continue the move smoothly over the pectoral muscles towards his stomach, taking your left hand away. Bend your knees to rock your body to the side if necessary to make this move easier, as it can be quite a stretch.

- Before your right hand reaches the end of the pectoral muscles (where you can feel that you 'fall off' a slight ridge onto your horse's abdomen), stretch your left arm out and put your left hand back at the starting position at the top of the muscle group, and start your effleurage all over again.

- I suggest around eight to ten seconds of effleurage through the pectoral muscles.

- Repeat this move six times, slowly but firmly, with as much pressure as feels right for you and your horse.

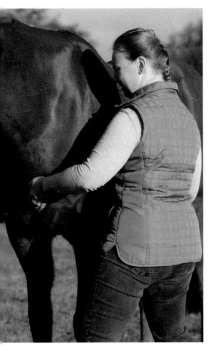

For the chest, effleurage is the only technique that I am suggesting to begin with. Stand beside him facing his shoulder, with your feet apart and your knees bent so that you can reach his chest and between his forelegs without having to bend your back.

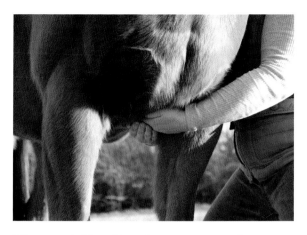

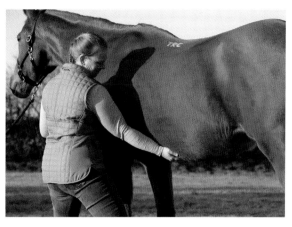

When your left hand is as far as you can reach between your horse's forelegs, place your right hand on top of your left hand and use it to continue the move smoothly over the *pectoral* muscles towards your horse's stomach, taking your left hand away.

Before your right hand reaches the end of the *pectoral* muscles, stretch your left arm out and put your left hand back at the starting position.

20. Repeat step 19 on the right side of your horse.

The whole body

21. To end the routine, stroke your horse gently and slowly over his whole body, as you did in step one.

To end the routine, stroke your horse gently and slowly over his whole body, as you did in step one.

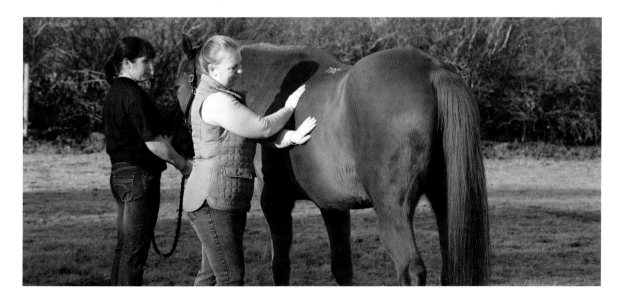

The end

22. To finish your massage, place one hand gently and lovingly on your horse's forehead, between his ears just where his forelock stops growing. If your horse prefers your hand on his neck, as some horses do, simply hold it there instead. Hold your hand still for a few seconds. Through your touch thank your horse for spending precious moments with you, and let him know how much you appreciate him. The results of his massage will often be quick to show, as he finds himself more comfortable and more flexible, and able to perform with less effort. The massage process should have been as enjoyable for you as it was for him, and you'll both already be looking forward to the next chance you have to spend time together.

To finish your massage, place one hand gently and lovingly on your horse's forehead, between his ears just where the forelock stops growing.

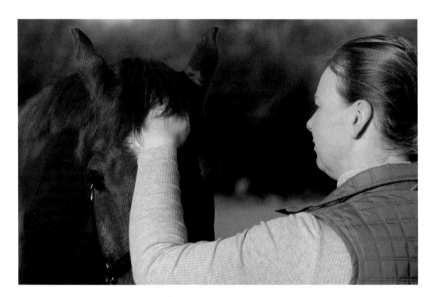

Helpful hints

Softly, softly

Many people have a tendency to press too hard when they're massaging the neck. Keep an eye on your horse's head and neck as you apply pressure along his neck from the shoulder towards the poll. If he moves his head away from your pressure, even a little, then you could be applying too much pressure. Try effleurage on your own arm or leg, or on a partner's back muscles, and see how lightly you can touch and yet still be felt and therefore have an effect. Massage does not always need heavy pressure to be effective. Even with a light touch you are affecting the nerve endings and therefore the nervous system of the entire body, as well as affecting the skin and much more.

Balance yourself

If your hand is hooked over your horse's withers when you are massaging, you will often subconsciously lean on that hand, which means that your horse has to brace to support you. Rest your hand lightly against his shoulder or ribcage to maintain connection, feel and awareness.

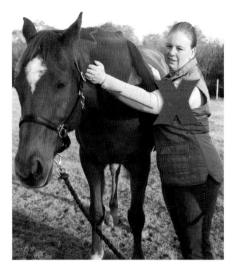

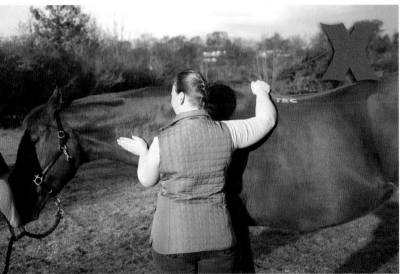

ABOVE Many people have a tendency to press too hard when massaging the neck. If your horse moves his head away from the pressure, even a little, then you could be applying too much pressure.

LEFT If your hand is hooked over your horse's withers when you are massaging, you will often subconsciously lean on that hand, which means that your horse has to brace to support you. Rest your hand lightly against his shoulder or ribcage to maintain connection, feel and awareness.

Slow down

In general, moving more slowly is more comfortable for your horse and more effective than moving quickly. Try working with a partner to get verbal feedback on different speeds of effleurage and compression. I suggest four seconds for many of the moves as a guide, but this is by no means a hard-and-fast rule. If you struggle to move slowly enough, count to yourself: try using the phrase 'one elephant, two elephant, three elephant, four elephant' (and remembering to pause between each 'elephant'!), or use your breathing to help you maintain consistency and calmness in your timing.

Start in the right place

It is much easier to be confident that you are massaging the correct area effectively if you take the time to draw the lines on the muscle, either using chalk or your finger. The most common mistake that I see is people not returning to the correct starting point, especially when working on the shoulder or the back. For some reason, a big percentage of students incorrectly 'move' their starting point for each of these moves to somewhere halfway along the horse's ribcage!

Be aware of your posture

Face your horse's side, and angle yourself towards his head or his tail as appropriate. At all times, stay aware of his expression and reactions. Have your feet wider apart if your horse is a pony, rather than bending down to massage him. Bend and straighten your knees to support the direction in which you are moving your hands (both in the effleurage and the compression), to lessen the impact or physical strain on your arms.

Use appropriate pressure

Practise to develop an intuitive awareness of your horse's skin and muscles, and his reaction to your massage. Try adjusting the pressure you use, and assess his reactions. A horse who is sore might flinch from your hand, or step away from you, or even pull a face or lift a hind leg to let you know he is sore. Sore muscle often feels hard, like a piece of board, and your horse's skin might twitch around the area you're working on. A horse who is comfortable will often lean into the pressure if it is slow enough. Pain-free muscle might feel more like Plasticine, with some give in it, and you can watch the ripple of muscle move in front of your hand like a wave as you apply effleurage.

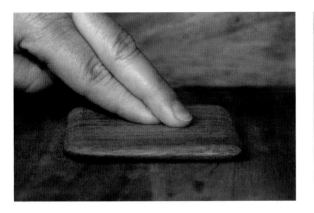 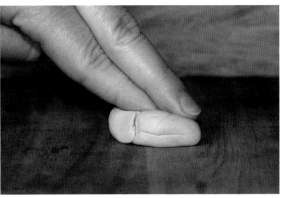

ABOVE LEFT Sore muscle often feels hard, like a piece of board.

ABOVE RIGHT Pain-free muscle might feel more like Plasticine, with some give in it, and you can watch the ripple of muscle move in front of your hand like a wave as you apply effleurage.

Stretch

One of the most common mistakes that I see in massaging the back and quarter muscles is people cutting the first line short. It's important that your hand goes all the way to reach your horse's back above where his coat changes direction. There are some very important muscles back there that are prone to being sore, and if you cut that line short, your horse will miss out on the benefit of massage in that area.

Enjoy

You'll either love or hate the kneading technique. If you love it, that's great – do more! If you hate it, either miss it out or do less. It takes a while to get the hang of the fact that different areas have different levels of 'skin slack'. Where your horse's skin is tight, there is very little movement in the 'twist' of the kneading move. Very little, however, is not the same as none at all, and you will still be having an effect. Your moves can be powerful without being big or dramatic. Try it on yourself; just the difference in skin slack from above your forearm to underneath your forearm should give you an idea of the variation.

One hand or both?

Most of the massage moves in this routine are performed with one hand. An exception to this is when you are working on the *trapezius* muscle, when both hands are used at the same time in harmony with each other.

Remember also to use both hands alternately for cupping, and to keep it very gentle. You can use the technique more firmly if it's safe to do so and if your horse enjoys it, but that can be harder on your body and might surprise your horse initially. Safety should always be your number one priority.

For a prompt section summing up the routine just described, see the back of the book.

4. Problem-solving

By reading this chapter you will:

- Gain an increased understanding of pain-related behaviours.

- Begin to relate anatomy to specific training or behavioural problems.

- Learn how to use massage techniques to address these anatomical areas in an attempt to resolve the problem.

Contributory factors to stiffness and soreness

Horses can suffer from stiffness and soreness in certain areas of their body. Often training difficulties or problem behaviours can be linked to a specific painful area. I find that every horse who is working hard from behind, whether that be through jumping, dressage, or racing for example, will have an increased chance of soreness through his quarters and his hamstrings. Every horse who lands heavily or works on hard ground, whether that be through jumping, racing, hacking on the roads, hunting, or driving, etc., has an increased chance of developing soreness through his forehand. Every horse who has, at some point, had a heavy-handed rider or an ill-fitting training aid, or has problems with his teeth, or has pulled back when tied up, has an increased chance of soreness through his neck. Every horse with a badly fitting saddle, or lameness in any leg (whether or not the lameness can be seen with the naked eye), will have an increased chance of soreness through his back and his chest.

Outside of this, specific training problems are commonly linked to specific musculoskeletal issues. This chapter discusses some of those problems, and the areas on which you might focus your massage techniques to improve your horse's performance and to help him work more easily and more correctly. It also gives you a 'checklist' of things to look for if you are concerned that your horse has soreness in a particular area of his body. Of course, this cannot be individualised in a book, and so I recommend that you seek advice from your vet, or from a well-qualified physical therapist (this includes physiotherapist, chiropractor or osteopath), saddler, dentist, farrier, or other qualified paraprofessional as appropriate.

Remember also that imbalances within your own body will have a powerful effect on your horse in his ridden work, so consider getting assessment and treatment for yourself from a qualified professional to determine whether you could be contributing to the problem.

Your horse communicates through his behaviour, including his body language. This means that if he is in pain, the only way he can show it is through his behaviour. I'm not just talking about the sort of pain that means that your horse says 'get off my back'. I'm also talking about the little niggling issues that mean he doesn't quite perform or behave as he should. Many horses are incredibly tolerant of what we perceive as pain, and seem keen to please their owner even if they are suffering themselves. Others are seemingly very intolerant to what we would categorise as mild pain, and as yet we cannot explain why this is so. Perhaps it's because the horse has pain that we can't yet detect. We can't always get it right, but if we try our hardest to listen to the horse then at least we are doing the best we can with the knowledge we have.

A general caveat with all the issues discussed in this 'problem-solving' chapter is that there are always many potential causes of a particular

Any horse will perform better if he is free from soreness and stiffness.

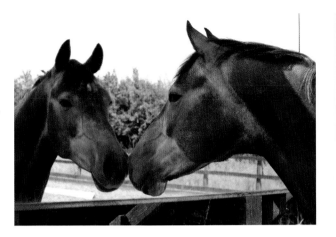

Your horse communicates with you through his behaviour.

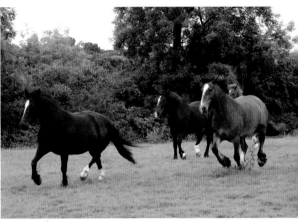

Struggling to pick up the correct canter lead can be a sign of pain.

problem or behaviour. Many are problems that require a professional to address, for example lameness, saddle fit, and foot balance. Others may have a behavioural element, or be contributed to by lack of knowledge or experience on the rider's part, and require the support of a good instructor or behaviourist. I have simply picked some issues that you can attempt to address with the massage techniques learned in this book. If your attempts are successful, then that's great, keep at it! If your attempts are unsuccessful, please, please seek professional help. Working as an equine behaviourist and chartered veterinary physiotherapist is incredibly rewarding, but can also be heart-breaking, and some horses are, often unknowingly on the part of their owner, mistreated through ignorance. Anger and frustration are purely the result of not knowing how to resolve a problem. All too often the choice of tools that are resorted to in addressing a particular training issue or behaviour is driven by these emotions. If more people could take the time to educate themselves in how to cause the required change in their horse's behaviour through fair and humane techniques, this could only benefit both horse and handler.

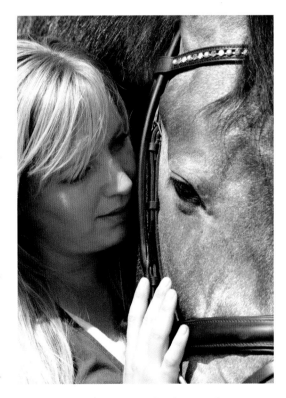

If more people would take the time to educate themselves in how to cause the required change in their horse's behaviour through fair and humane techniques, this could only benefit both horse and handler.

Checklists

The neck

If the answer to any of these questions is 'yes', I recommend that you contact a professional to assess your horse more thoroughly.

- If you run the pads of your fingers slowly and firmly down the middle of or along the bottom of the neck muscles, does your horse tense up against the pressure or flinch away from you? (This is a different feeling from him moving his head away from you because of the pressure you're applying.) Your fingers should sink into the muscle like into Plasticine.

- If you ask your horse to stand still and bend his head to the left, and then bend his head to the right, does he bend further or more easily in one direction than the other? Does he resist more one way than the other?

- Is your horse head-shy or spooky?

- Do you have difficulty putting the bridle on, or does he pull back when tied up?

Could your horse be stiff or sore through his neck?

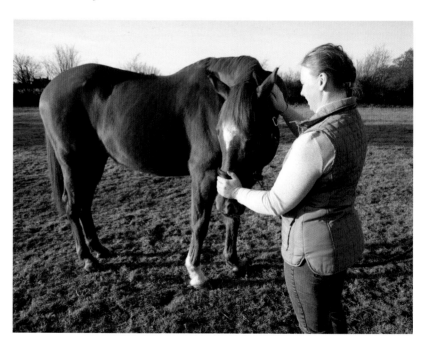

- Has your horse suffered from dental issues?

- Is your horse heavy in your hand or strong in his ridden work?

As I mentioned before, there are myriad reasons why your horse might demonstrate any of these problems, one of these being 'lameness'. Lameness is very difficult to define, but it will almost always involve asymmetry of movement, in that the right side of the horse moves differently from the left. Sometimes this can't be seen by the naked eye, and the inexperienced eye can easily miss mild lameness. If your horse is sore in one or more legs, that soreness will affect the way he moves. In relation to bend for example, if your horse is sore through his right fore, he may feel more stiff or resistant to the right because he will try to avoid putting extra weight through the sore leg. If this were the case, then you would need to work with your vet to address the root cause before any massage would be effective in relieving the stiffness.

One aspect on which you can have a beneficial effect and that often causes stiffness to one side is tension and soreness at the poll. Horses who have pulled back when tied up are classic examples of this (and their action may have triggered other problems as well). Usually I find that these horses are stiff in the same direction as the side of the poll that is

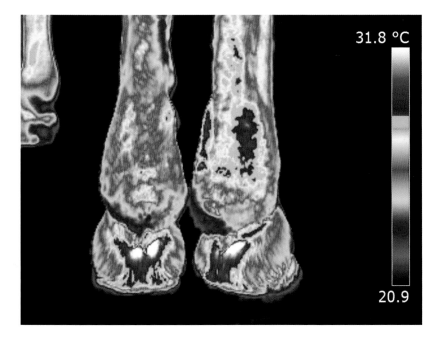

31.8 °C

20.9

If your horse is sore in one leg, that soreness will affect the way he moves.
(Image courtesy Jackie Lockett)

most sore. You can help to relieve this with massage, and therefore help your horse to become more flexible and even in his work.

In-depth massage

Concentrate on massaging your horse's neck muscle as discussed in the previous chapter, but use at least double the number of effleurage and compression moves. Then use cross-fibre friction just behind his ear, in the soft area between the back of his ear and the front of the bone at the top of his neck. Work as softly as needed but as firmly as tolerated, for at least a minute (longer if necessary) until you feel any resistance in the muscle soften under your fingers. Go back to effleurage and compression along his neck muscle as described in the routine, again at least doubling the numbers of each move.

Next, stand by your horse's shoulder with your back to him and gently guide his head around towards you until he is 'hugging' you. Ask him to hold this position for around one to two minutes. He must hold his head there willingly with a relaxed posture, rather than resisting against you. If he's finding it difficult, don't ask him to bend as far, or for as long. Repeat, asking him to bend around you to his other side, again holding

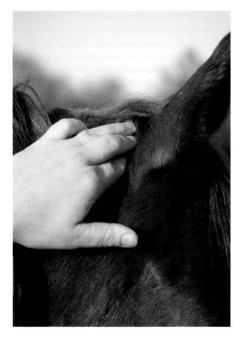

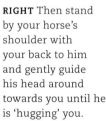

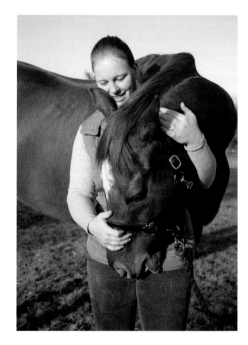

LEFT Use cross-fibre friction to relieve stiffness or soreness at the poll.

RIGHT Then stand by your horse's shoulder with your back to him and gently guide his head around towards you until he is 'hugging' you.

for one to two minutes. Do this three times on each side. You should find that, by the third time, your horse bends more easily than he did when you started. Then once more carry out your 'neck' massage techniques of effleurage and compression to stimulate circulation and lymphatic drainage and to offer pain relief.

The shoulder

If the answer to any of these questions is 'yes', I recommend that you contact a professional to assess your horse more thoroughly.

- If you press into your horse's muscles just in front of or just behind his shoulder-blade, does he tighten up against you, flinch, or dip away from the pressure? Your fingers should sink into the muscle as though they were sinking into Plasticine, without any adverse reaction from your horse.

- Does your horse trip often?

- Does your horse knock the occasional fence down without any apparent reason?

- Does your horse trot more freely on soft ground than he does on hard ground?

- Does your horse have an unexpectedly short, choppy, 'pony' stride?

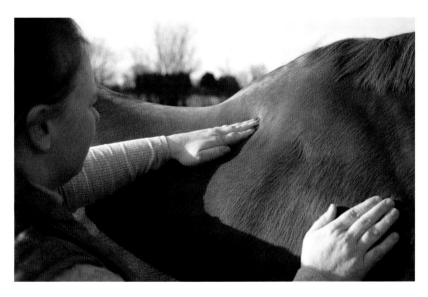

Could your horse be stiff or sore through his shoulder?

Many horses are restricted from achieving their full potential because their length of stride is affected by soreness through their shoulders and their chest. This can lead to tripping, and poor jumping performance, and can dramatically reduce dressage marks and the ability to gallop at speed. (Of course there are plenty of other reasons for a horse to shorten his stride, including poor saddle fit, poor foot balance, and lameness.)

Relieving stiffness and soreness through your horse's shoulder could improve length of stride.

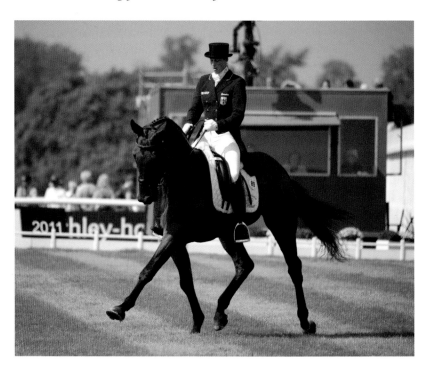

In-depth massage

The most effective massage work that you can do to address this is to work on the neck, the shoulder, the back and the chest. And, of course, once you've helped the front end of your horse to move more freely, you then need to massage his quarters so that he can work better from behind! I discuss neck, back, chest and quarters in other sections of this chapter, so here I'm going to talk about massaging the shoulder with regards to problem-solving.

You will know from Chapter 2 that the *trapezius* muscle is involved in the movement of your horse's shoulder-blade, and that movement of his shoulder-blade is linked to the movement of his foreleg. It is also involved in pulling his withers down towards his shoulder-blades (the opposite of what you are looking for when he's working correctly), and so must be pain-free in order for your horse to 'lift through his withers'. It's essential that the shoulder-blades are able to move freely in relation to the neck, ribcage and withers in order for your horse to achieve his optimum length of stride.

Begin by using the massage techniques described in the massage routine: effleurage, compression, and more effleurage. Next, feel around the top of your horse's shoulder-blade. See if you can feel the front of his shoulder-blade where it meets his neck muscle, the top of his shoulder-blade below his withers, and the back of his shoulder-blade where the front of his saddle would sit. Use cross-fibre friction to work slowly into the area around the top of his shoulder-blade within his *trapezius* muscle. Work around the outside of the edge of his shoulder-blade, not over the surface of it. Then move your fingers up to the withers and use slow cross-fibre friction close to his spine. Start along the side of your horse's dorsal spinous processes, from as far towards the top of his withers as possible, and continue to a point somewhere around the middle of his back. Finish with your original techniques of effleurage, compression and effleurage, and then repeat the entire process on the other side of your horse.

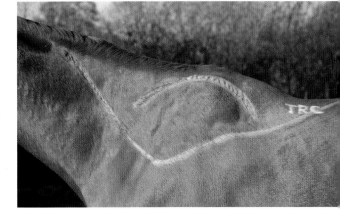

Use cross-fibre friction to work slowly into the area around the top of the shoulder-blade within the *trapezius* muscle, to relieve stiffness and soreness in this area.

You and your horse will dictate the amount of pressure that you use in your cross-fibre friction. Be careful to stay slow in your massaging; it's easy to get carried away. Try to forget about the stresses of daily life. Use your breathing to maintain a rhythm in your work, and to focus on yourself and your horse.

The back

If the answer to any of these questions is 'yes', I recommend that you contact a professional to assess your horse more thoroughly.

- If you run your fingers *slowly* along the top of your horse's spine with a firm pressure, does he twitch/shiver/dip away from your hand? Please note that if you run your finger *quickly* along his back muscle,

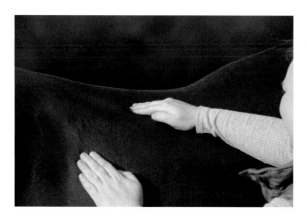

Could your horse be stiff or sore through his back?

you will elicit a reflex that causes him to dip his back away from you, however, this reflex should not be elicited by a slow movement. If in doubt, seek the advice of a professional.

- Does your horse seem sore or pull faces when you groom him, or when you rug him up?

- Do you have difficulty getting your horse to stand square, either ridden or from the ground?

- Does your horse pull a face or move away from you when you go to put his saddle on?

- Does your horse have difficulty standing still for you to get on, or 'put his back up' or move off in a hurry once you're on?

- Does your horse have a tendency to rush, or to be unexpectedly lazy when ridden?

- Does your horse buck, rear or nap?

- Does your horse become more agitated or difficult towards the end of a ride, either in the school or out hacking?

Any of these issues could potentially be related to back pain. As always, there are plenty of other possible causes of each of these behaviours, and there are also lots of causes of back pain. For example, it's well-documented that lameness can lead to back pain, and most people are aware that poor saddle fit will make your horse sore through his back. Skeletal issues such as arthritis in the spine and kissing spine are also likely to lead to back pain.

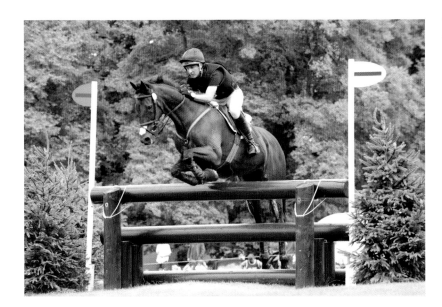

Your horse needs to be pain-free to work correctly through his back.

As I mentioned in the early part of this chapter, it's great to have a go and see if you can help your horse through massage. However, if the situation does not seem to be improving, I strongly recommend that you ask for help from a professional. Sometimes manual therapy is not enough to overcome the problem, and allowing your horse to be as pain-free as possible should be a priority, especially when we ask our horses not only to accept the weight of a rider, but also to perform to the best of their ability whilst carrying that rider.

In-depth massage

Depending on the root cause of the problem, you may be able to go a long way to alleviating any pain that there might be in your horse's back by using massage. Part of the solution is to increase the amount of time that you spend working on that area. Start by using the techniques discussed in the massage routine: effleurage, compression, and more effleurage. You will remember that, in the routine explained earlier, you drew three lines on your horse's back, and worked along those three lines. If you suspect a problem in your horse's back and are trying to ease pain or stiffness, you could increase the number of lines that you work along, so that you cover more of the area, still working within the rectangle that you drew to represent the *longissimus dorsi* muscle. You could also add another two lines, one that goes straight along the top of the rectangle (just off the spine), and another that goes straight along the bottom of the rectangle (along the top of the ribcage). Use at least three sets of effleurage along each line, then three sets of compression, and then a further three sets of effleurage.

Next, use cross-fibre friction. Use a level of pressure that is accepted by your horse, and that is comfortable for your body. Work initially along the top of your horse's ribcage, using the cross-fibre friction technique every centimetre or so to release any tension in his muscles. Work from the front to the rear of your horse's back. Keep going past the end of his ribcage, at the same level as the top of his ribcage, until you get to where his coat changes direction at the bony protuberance that's known as his point of hip. This will mean that you cover not only the muscles that span the length of his back, but you also have an effect on the important abdominal muscles and some of the muscles that control his pelvis. Then use the same process working along the side of your horse's spine, again every centimetre or so from front to rear. If you come across a spot that feels tighter than the areas around it, or that causes your horse to tense up against you, work for longer on that area until it softens under your fingers.

Finish helping to improve your horse's comfort through his back by returning to your original techniques of effleurage, compression, and

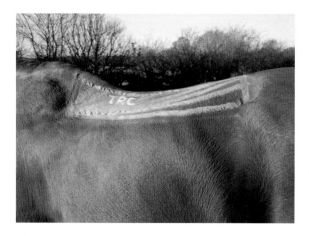

If you suspect a problem in your horse's back and are trying to ease pain or stiffness, you could increase the number of lines that you work along, so that you cover more of the area.

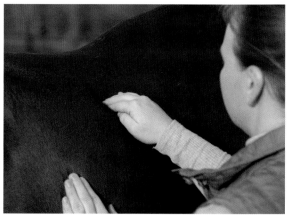

You could also use cross-fibre friction, at a level of pressure that is accepted by your horse, and that is comfortable for your body.

more effleurage. You may find that your horse's muscles feel softer and suppler, and he might respond to the changes by relaxing, yawning or stretching.

The quarters

If the answer to any of these questions is 'yes', I recommend that you contact a professional to assess your horse more thoroughly.

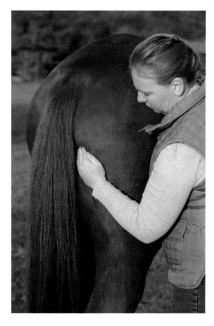

- If you stroke slowly but firmly either up or down your horse's hamstring muscles either side of his tail, do you feel those muscles twitching and tightening up against the pressure, or does your horse swish his tail or lift his leg?

- If you press firmly with the pads of your fingers against the hair in lines from your horse's hip to his spine, does he round his back or dip his back down? (Keep an eye on the middle of his back as well as the area just in front of your fingers.)

- Does your horse struggle to track up (to place his hind feet in or in front of the hoofprint left by his forefeet)?

- Does your horse move with his quarters to one side in his ridden work?

Could your horse be stiff or sore through his quarters?

- Does your horse refuse fences for no apparent reason?

- Does your horse find it difficult to hold his hind feet up for the farrier?

The quarters contain a huge bulk of muscle. It can be daunting trying to affect this area with massage, because there is a tendency to believe that you have to use enormous levels of pressure to work deep enough to make a difference. Because of the way the body is designed, however, even the effects of light touch are transferred deep within the body. Also, it might seem incredible, but through massaging the quarters (including the hamstrings) you can relieve tension in the neck and poll, and vice versa. As always, bear in mind that professional input may be required to help your horse overcome his difficulties. However, the amount of muscle in the quarters makes this an ideal area for you to improve with massage.

In-depth massage

The massage routine initially discussed, involving drawing three lines on your horse's quarters, and then using effleurage, kneading, cupping and more effleurage, is helpful in this region. One suggestion is to draw more lines to work along on his quarters, so that you cover more of the area with your massage techniques. You can then use not only effleurage, but also compression along these lines. In particular, using compression towards the front of your horse's quarters through the *gluteus medius* muscle can be very effective. Use the compression technique every couple of centimetres, working slowly with a level of pressure that is comfortable for both you and your horse.

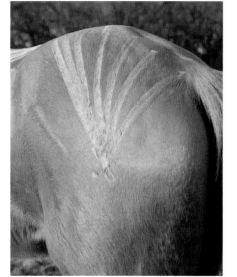

One suggestion is to draw more lines to work along in this region, so that you cover more of the quarters with your massage techniques.

To further improve the benefit that you can offer your horse, I recommend using more of the kneading technique through his hamstring muscles. Work gently, so that your horse doesn't feel the need to demonstrate a pain reaction whilst you are standing near his hind leg. In particular, concentrate around the top of the *semitendinosus* muscle, between your horse's seat bone and the top of his tail and the area just below his seat bone. If he's relaxed enough and it's safe to do so, work on the inside of the muscle in these areas as well as on the outside. As with your other techniques, increase the amount of time that you work here, up to five minutes or so on the left of your horse, and the same on the right.

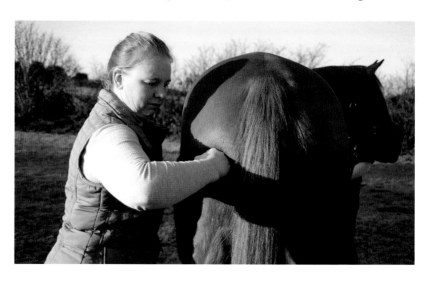

To further improve the benefit that you can offer your horse, I recommend using more of the kneading technique through the hamstring muscles.

The *biceps femoris* muscle is often tight and sore close to the stifle area. This is a region that can be particularly sensitive, so only work here if you are safe to do so. Gentle cupping is an easy and effective technique to use here if your horse accepts it. Often, working with one hand is easier than working with both as you get closer to the stifle. Find a steady rhythm that feels right, and gently cup from your horse's hip towards his stifle. This softly mobilises the muscle right through to the inside of his hind leg. Continue for at least three minutes to allow the muscle to react and soften to the mobilisation. Finish by using effleurage to complete your in-depth massage work to your horse's quarters.

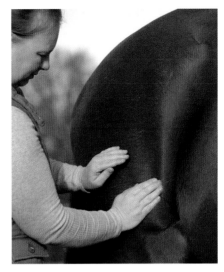

Gentle cupping around the stifle area, if safe to do, softly mobilises the muscle right through to the inside of the hind leg.

The chest

If the answer to any of these questions is 'yes', I recommend that you contact a professional to assess your horse more thoroughly.

- When you stroke your horse on his chest or between his forelegs, does he show displeasure?

- Is your horse ticklish to groom in his girth area?

- When you fasten your horse's rug at the front, does he try to bite you or hold on to the stable door with his teeth?

- Does your horse 'blow up' when you do his girth up, or threaten to bite or kick?

- Do you have to lunge your horse before you feel he's safe to ride?

- Is your horse 'cold-backed', or does he rush off when you first get on?

The pectoral muscles and the surrounding area are probably uncomfortable in the horses that I treat more so than any other area. The relief that your horse can experience when the soreness and tension in this area is eased we can only imagine to be immense, with corresponding improvements in both behaviour and performance. Of course, as with every other area of the body, there are many causes of problems in this area, and the issue cannot always be resolved through massage. One important example of this is gastric ulcers, which can cause reactivity throughout the girth region, including through the pectoral muscles. If you suspect that your horse might be suffering from gastric ulcers, you should contact your vet for advice.

In-depth massage

You will remember that, in the massage routine, you used only effleurage in your horse's chest area. This is because so many horses are sore in this area. More in-depth massage techniques can cause a very sore horse to tighten up against your touch, which can be detrimental rather than beneficial. Often, the best way of helping relieve this soreness is simply to increase the amount of effleurage that you offer. You might even spend five or ten minutes each side, working softly through the horse's pectoral muscles in a steady rhythm until he is less reactive to your touch, or until his muscles feel softer under your fingers. If you can repeat this on a daily basis for a week or a month, there is a strong chance that you will notice a significant change in your horse's attitude and ability to work.

Often the best way of helping relieve soreness in the chest region is simply to increase the amount of effleurage that you offer.

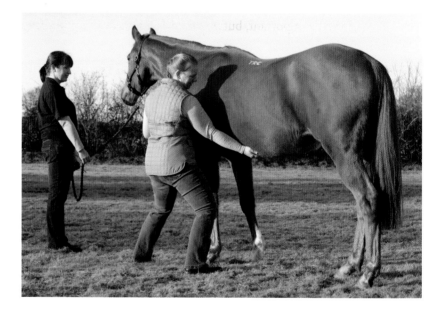

Although effleurage is the most prevalent technique to use in the chest area, sometimes it's helpful to work more precisely and include cross-fibre friction in your massage of this region. Perhaps surprisingly, I would recommend starting by working more deeply through the shoulder region, as described earlier in this chapter. Then go back to the chest region and see if your horse is more comfortable here, since the two are closely linked. Then use cross-fibre friction through his pectoral muscles by working either side of his breast bone (sternum). You can find his breast bone most easily at the front of your horse, low down in the middle of his chest. You can feel the hard bone as opposed to the soft muscle either side of and above the breast bone, and it continues centrally between his legs and part-way along his midline.

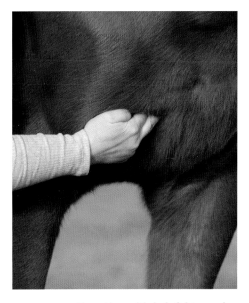

Sometimes it's helpful to work more precisely and include cross-fibre friction in your massage of the chest region.

Staying aware of your posture so that you minimise the stress through your own body, work along each side of your horse's sternum from front towards back, using the cross-fibre friction technique every centimetre or so. If you come to an area that seems tighter than expected, or causes him to react adversely, work gently using cross-fibre friction to relieve the problem. Remember that your speed of movement (slower is generally better), and the length of time you apply the technique for (longer is generally better) are important, but you do not need to use a heavy level of pressure.

As always, finish your massage work with effleurage, as described in the massage routine.

5. Frequently Asked Questions

In this chapter you will find the answers to the following questions:

1. How often should I massage my horse?

2. How long should the massage routine last?

3. What will massage do for my horse?

4. What does a knot feel like?

5. Does it matter which direction I perform the massage move in?

6. You've explained about cross-fibre friction, why is it not in the basic routine?

7. Should I massage before or after exercise?

8. Is my horse to young/too old for massage?

9. Can I massage my pregnant mare?

10. My horse doesn't seem to enjoy his massage – what can I do?

11. What do I do if my horse seems sore?

12. What research is there to support massage as a therapy?

13. My physiotherapist/osteopath/chiropractor/massage therapist has explained that they need to contact my vet before they can treat my horse. Please can you explain why?

14. What is the difference between physiotherapy, osteopathy and chiropractic?

15. Where can I find more answers?

1. How often should I massage my horse?

You can massage your horse as often as you like. The most important factor is to listen to the horse. If he is telling you that he is enjoying his massage then all is well and good. If he is telling you that he is not enjoying his massage, then take the time to work out whether you need to adapt your technique, or whether he is in need of assessment and treatment from a qualified professional. Massage reduces pain and stiffness and improves performance. Therefore it can only be beneficial, as long as you have ruled out any reasons why he should not be massaged – see the Contraindications section in Chapter 3.

I tend to suggest a 'gold standard' schedule whereby you massage your horse once a week, a 'recommended' schedule of once a month, or a 'must have' schedule of once every three months. If you have an equine professional working with your horse, such as a veterinarian, physiotherapist, osteopath, chiropractor or qualified massage therapist, they will advise you how best to support the work that they have done or are doing.

The 'gold standard' once-a-week massage will really enable you to get to know your horse well, and he will enjoy to his treatment. Many riders I meet would like to ride every day but feel that it is only fair to give the horse one day off a week. This day off is the ideal time to offer a weekly massage. You will develop a feel for what is normal in terms of muscle tension and development for your horse, and this will allow you to recognise when something develops that is not normal. You can then address this appropriately before it becomes a problem that your horse demonstrates to you through his behaviour.

Massage can be used as a preventative therapy, to maintain good health, muscle function and flexibility, as much as a technique to improve performance. This is best achieved through regular treatment. Remember that your horse is an athlete, and should be treated as such. This is obvious when you think about competition horses, but also applies to horse who simply hack out – they are effectively hiking with a backpack! We wouldn't expect successful human athletes to compete without regular therapy, so why should we expect that of our horses?

Often a rider will demand far more in terms of fitness from their horse than they will demand from themselves. Time and again I see riders tacking their horse up in the stable, bringing him out into the yard and getting straight on. We have been taught to think of warming up as something we do when we are riding the horse, but think about the effort that the horse's muscles have to use to carry the weight of the rider. Would it perhaps be fairer to do some 'warming up' before we even get on?

Massaging your horse the 'recommended' once a month means that you keep an eye on his physical wellbeing on a regular basis, as well as giving your horse some quality time. It's easy to get overwhelmed with all that goes on in our lives. Instead of time with our horse being a pleasure, it can become a chore; something that needs to be 'fitted in' around everything else. A monthly 'pamper session' is a great way of giving something back to your horse in return for all that he gives to you. To massage effectively you need 'quiet time', you have to focus on yourself and your horse and forget about the outside world, and that can be as beneficial for you as it is for your horse.

The three-monthly 'must have' can be thought of as a regular 'MOT' for your horse. It gives you a chance to check him over thoroughly for any signs of stiffness or soreness, and to assess whether he would benefit from professional therapy of any kind. You could fit this in, for example, every other time he was due to be shod.

It can be useful to take a photograph of your horse each time you massage him, so that you have a record of how he has changed from the outside, if at all, and photographic documentation to look back on if you have any concerns.

It can be useful to take a photograph of your horse each time you massage him, so that you have a record of how he has changed from the outside, if at all, and photographic documentation to look back on if you have any concerns.

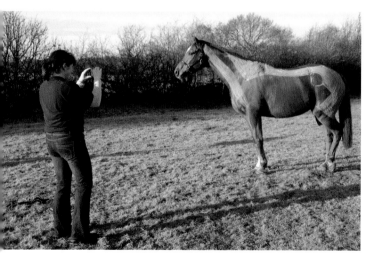

If you are addressing a particular problem with your horse and working alongside an equine professional, they will advise how often you should work with him, and if there are any particular areas to focus on. There are occasions when massage every day would be beneficial, and occasions when massage might be harmful rather than beneficial. Perhaps you could show them this book, and the anatomy and massage techniques taught in it, so that they are aware of the knowledge that you have and can target your input more effectively.

2. How long should the massage routine last?

The massage can last as long as is right for you and your horse. If you follow closely the routine I've described in this book then it will take an average of around forty-five minutes to one hour. However, if you use either fewer or more compressions in each move (carried out on the neck, shoulder and back), you can lessen or increase this time considerably. You may find that your horse prefers you to work a little faster, or more slowly. Once you are confident following the routine with the suggested number of moves for each technique, you may find that you and/or your horse prefer one technique more than another, and you could choose to do more of this particular technique and less of others.

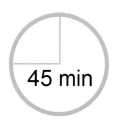

The massage can last as long as is right for you and your horse. If you follow closely the routine I've described in this book then it will take an average of around forty-five minutes to one hour.

Adding on extras as described in Chapter 4 will also increase the time that your massage takes. Some horses find it difficult to stand still for this length of time, and so you may decide to break the routine down into more manageable chunks, perhaps working with the neck, shoulders and chest one day, then the back and quarters another day. This can be particularly relevant for youngsters. Some horses find it difficult initially to relax into the massage, and you might find that they accept it more readily if you break it down into sections, or do less of each move for the first few massages. It can seem almost as though they need time to get used to the fact that you're wanting to help them feel better, since they've got so used to feeling the way they do, being independent and looking after themselves.

3. What will massage do for my horse?

The benefits of massage have been shown scientifically to include pain relief, reduced anxiety and depression, reduced blood pressure, and reduced heart rate. It is believed that massage might also stimulate the release of endorphins and serotonin, reduce scar tissue, increase the flow of lymph, have an effect on the release of hormones, and improve sleep. Because of the nature of massage as a manual therapy, it is difficult to develop 'sham' treatments, because even light touch is still a form of massage. It is impossible for the therapist not to know that they are treating the patient, and difficult for the patient not to realise that they are receiving a massage, both of which are required for double-blind clinical trials. This means that it's difficult to produce 'gold standard' research on massage.

4. What does a knot feel like?

A 'knot' is an area within the muscle that has contracted, and for some reason has not relaxed again. Think of the knot like a twisted tangle of muscle fibres, like a knotted rope, and this is what you can feel underneath the skin. It is not normal for any muscle to stay contracted for prolonged periods, and the contraction causes a restriction of blood flow to the area. This means fewer nutrients to the affected part of the muscle, and poor removal of waste.

The best way to discover what a 'knot' feels like is to try to find one on a friend. The easiest place is usually around the top of their shoulder-blade. Your friend will be able to tell you when you find the 'knot' because when you apply strong pressure it will feel different from the tissue around it. It might feel more painful, or like a dull ache, or the classic 'it hurts but it's a good hurt' kind of feeling.

Try hiding a lock of hair under a piece of paper, then closing your eyes and feeling over the top of the piece of paper to find the hair. This will give you an idea of feeling through the skin for a 'knot'. Increase your sensitivity by putting another piece of paper on top of the first, and then another, and seeing how many pieces of paper you can put on top before you lose the ability to feel that lock of hair.

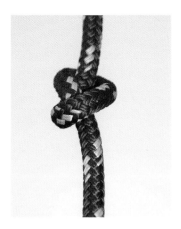

A 'knot' is an area within the muscle that has contracted, and for some reason has not relaxed again. Think of it like a twisted tangle of muscle fibres, like a knotted rope.

5. Does it matter which direction I perform the massage move in?

Often people are confused as to whether or not it's okay to massage against their horse's hair, or whether they need to be massaging towards the heart (as in lymphatic drainage massage). If you are not working as a professional massage therapist, and your goal is a holistic whole body approach to reducing stiffness and pain, then the direction in which you massage is unlikely to alter the effect of the massage in this particular routine. There are many cases in which the direction of massage does matter, but this is not one of them. My hope is that, as you become more confident using the massage techniques, then you'll experiment to find what works best for you and your horse.

6. You've explained about cross-fibre friction, why is it not in the basic routine?

The basic massage routine includes effleurage, compression, kneading, and cupping. These are the techniques that I recommend you use on a regular basis with your horse to offer a general wellbeing massage for comfort, health and performance. If, whilst massaging your horse, you find an area that you feel requires a deeper technique to release tension, you could try using cross-fibre frictions as described under The Chest in Chapter 4.

7. Should I massage before or after exercise?

Whether to massage your horse before or after exercise is a great question, and there are good arguments for both sides, as both are beneficial. Personally, I favour massaging your horse before exercise. The reason for this is that, since massage reduces pain and stiffness and improves performance, the horse who has been massaged before work will perform more easily. This means that you will have a more enjoyable ride and will offer him more reward and less correction. We all know that reward will encourage your horse to offer more, therefore the ride is more enjoyable, and so on. If he is able to use his body more correctly, he will perform the movements more easily and be compensating less through muscles struggling to cope with the work, effectively giving himself his own physical therapy by working more symmetrically. This continuous cycle of improvement can only be good for horse and rider, not only physically but also mentally and emotionally.

Since massage reduces pain and stiffness and improves performance, the horse who has been massaged before work will perform more easily.

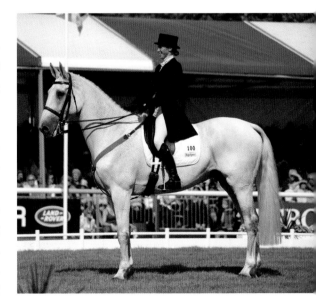

Massaging your horse after you work him, however, also has many benefits. During the session your horse's body will release waste products that need to be removed by the lymphatic drainage system, and massage stimulates this system. Microscopic soft tissue injuries will have happened; maybe slight bruising under his saddle, or a tweak in his fetlock as he slipped on a corner, or a resistance to the rein causing tension in his poll and down his neck. Even a horse working

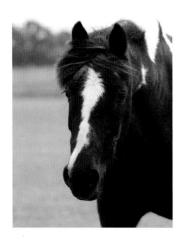

You can massage a horse at any age. The mare in this photo is 28 years old.

with no resistance to the rider will experience tissue breakdown as he builds strength. Massage also promotes circulation, which carries the nutrients to these areas to enable healing. And so massaging your horse after his work will lead to improved recovery from that session.

8. Is my horse to young/too old for massage?

No! You can massage a horse at any age. If your horse is very young then he may find it difficult to stand still for too long, and you can adapt your routine accordingly, perhaps by just working on the shoulder area one day, and the back another day, for example. If your horse is very old, massage is an excellent way of maintaining his good health.

9. Can I massage my pregnant mare?

This is something that you need to discuss with your veterinarian, as there may be contraindications to massage during certain stages of pregnancy.

10. My horse doesn't seem to enjoy his massage – what can I do?

Usually the answer is to work more slowly. Preference for speed and pressure levels is very individual. It is also important to work in a way that is physically comfortable for you, because otherwise your tension will be felt by your horse. Try taking six or eight seconds to do each move, rather than four seconds. Experiment with pressing harder or more softly.

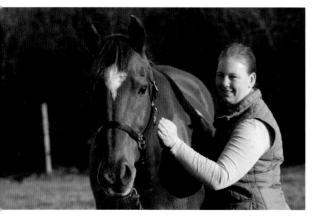

If your horse doesn't seem to be enjoying his massage, work more slowly.

You could try massaging with a body brush or with a rubber curry comb instead of with your hands, and see if the different sensation improves your horse's acceptance of the techniques. Some horses will take three or four massage sessions before they understand what you are doing for them and begin to enjoy it.

Bear in mind that, when you are initially learning the techniques and the routine, the massage that you give is likely to be stilted and without as much understanding and emotion as there will be once you get more confident. Give yourself time to get used to the massage and be tolerant of any mistakes you make, and ask the same of your horse.

It could be that your horse is sore and so your touch is painful. If in doubt, call a professional and ask them to assess your horse as an individual.

11. What do I do if my horse seems sore?

Your first port of call should be your vet, who will assess your horse and advise the best course of action. You can find your local chartered animal physiotherapist at www.acpat.co.uk, and they will work in conjunction with your vet to help you and your horse. Ask your physiotherapist to give you some exercises that you can continue with once they have left (if appropriate) and take note of any advice in relation to how soon after treatment you should ride your horse and whether he would benefit from further treatments. It may be that they can suggest specific areas on which you should concentrate your massage techniques to best improve your horse's comfort levels.

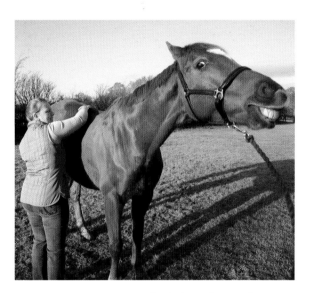

A physiotherapist may be able to suggest specific areas where you can concentrate your massage techniques to best improve your horse's comfort levels.

12. What research is there to support massage as a therapy?

More research is carried out into treatment of musculoskeletal pain and improvement in performance through massage in human beings than in horses, for various reasons. We tend to assume that the effects for horses are similar to those for human beings. In the human field, massage has been shown many times to be effective, especially when combined with exercise and advice. Importantly to you, as a reader who is not experienced in massage, research also shows massage to be safe.

In the UK, the National Institute for Health and Clinical Excellence (NICE) is an independent organisation responsible for providing national guidance on promoting good health and preventing ill health (in human beings). NICE offers research-based guidance on a variety of health topics. In its guidance on the treatment of low back pain (2011), NICE recommends 'offering a course of manual therapy ... comprising up to a maximum of nine sessions over a period of up to 12 weeks'. NICE goes on to state that the manual therapies reviewed were spinal manipulation, spinal mobilisation and massage.

A group of scientists called the Cochrane Group review all available evidence on a particular subject (again in the human field rather than the equine). In June 2010, a Cochrane review was published regarding the effectiveness of massage for low back pain. The group found that 'No serious adverse events were reported by any patient in the included studies.' Massage, defined as soft tissue manipulation using hands or a mechanical device, was shown to be more effective than several other forms of treatment when combined with exercise and education. Their conclusion was that massage might be beneficial for patients with short- and long-term non-specific low back pain, especially when combined with exercises and education.

In February 2011, when reviewing the effectiveness of massage for mechanical neck disorders, the same group stated that: 'Results showed that massage is safe and any side effects were temporary and benign.' However, they found that there was such a wide range of massage techniques used in the studies that they couldn't get an overall picture of the effectiveness of massage or draw firm conclusions for its effectiveness in improving neck pain or function.

A 2008 study assessing the effects of massage, chiropractic, bute, field rest and ridden work on horses with no known problems found that massage was the only treatment to consistently lead to an improvement right from day one.

Moving on to horses, in 2008 a study was published in the *Equine Veterinary Journal* (and reported in *Horse and Hound*) demonstrating the effectiveness of equine massage for decreasing pain. A pressure algometer (a device validated in the human field for measuring pain thresholds) was used to assess objectively the level of pressure a horse would accept before an 'avoidance reaction' was shown. The horses were then divided into treatment groups (receiving chiropractic, massage, bute, field rest, or ridden work) and treated, before being assessed again using the pressure algometer over the next few days. Massage and chiropractic were clearly shown to have a greater effect on pain thresholds than the other treatment options, with massage being the only treatment to consistently lead to an improvement right from day one.

In November 2010 a study was reported in the *Equine Veterinary Journal* entitled 'The relationship between massage to the equine caudal hind limb muscles and hind limb protraction'. The authors Carolyn Hill and Tracy Crook noted that 'massage is widely used in physiotherapy'. This study involved eight horses randomly assigned to two groups of four. One group received massage to the hamstring muscles for thirty minutes, with the other group receiving a sham treatment. After seven days, the groups were swapped and the first group received thirty minutes of sham treatment, whilst the second group received thirty minutes of massage to the hamstring muscles. Hind limb range of movement, specifically length of stride and the ability of the horse to have his hind limb stretched forward underneath him, was measured before and after each intervention. The results showed that this range of movement was increased following massage, and the study concluded that massage could potentially play a valuable role in rehabilitation or performance improvement. This research supports the use of massage with horses and, as a safe technique, it is something that you as an owner, with appropriate guidance, can do for your own horse.

13. My physiotherapist/osteopath/chiropractor/massage therapist has explained that they need to contact my vet before they can treat my horse. Please can you explain why?

This is a legal matter and is in the interests of ensuring that only people qualified to do so treat animals. The Veterinary Surgery (Exemptions) Order 1962 allows for the treatment of animals by 'physiotherapy', provided that the animal has first been seen by a veterinary surgeon who has diagnosed the condition and decided that it should be treated by physiotherapy under his/her direction. 'Physiotherapy' is interpreted in this case as including all kinds of manipulative therapy. It therefore includes osteopathy and chiropractic but would not, for example, include acupuncture or aromatherapy. (Royal College of Veterinary Surgeons Guide To Professional Conduct, section 2F: Treatment of animals by non-veterinary surgeons, September 2011.)

Importantly within this legislation, there is a requirement for all equine physical therapists, whether massage therapists or physiotherapists, to work under veterinary referral. You should expect to be asked by your therapist either to contact your vet yourself to gain this referral, or to be asked for your vet's details so that the therapist can contact your vet directly.

14. What is the difference between physiotherapy, osteopathy and chiropractic?

Since a question I'm commonly asked is 'What is the difference between physiotherapy, osteopathy and chiropractic?', I've included here for you a brief description not only of physiotherapy, but also of osteopathy and chiropractic work in relation to animals.

What is physiotherapy?

'Physiotherapy helps restore movement and function to as near normal as possible when someone is affected by injury, illness or by developmental or other disability.' (Chartered Society of Physiotherapy website 2011.)

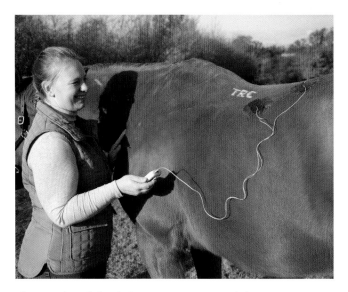

The practice of physiotherapy covers manual therapy, electrotherapy and exercise therapy. TENS is an example of electrotherapy as a treatment technique.

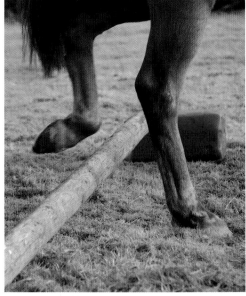

Exercise is a well-proven treatment technique.

Physiotherapy covers a wide range of treatments, including manual therapy, electrotherapy and exercise therapy, and massage is a core skill. The physiotherapist aims to reduce pain, benefit healing, and improve performance. Chartered physiotherapists have specialist knowledge of anatomy and biomechanics, physiology and pathology, and use detailed assessment to tailor treatments to each animal, its condition and the stage of the problem.

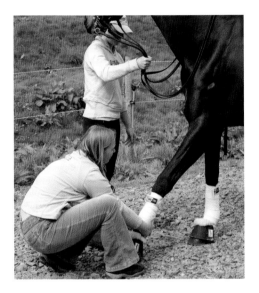
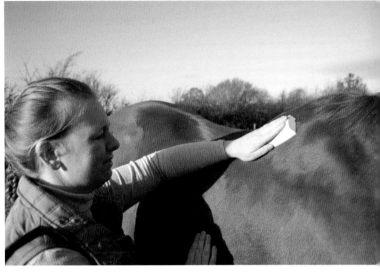

ABOVE LEFT Your physiotherapist might use stretches as a treatment for your horse.

ABOVE RIGHT Chartered physiotherapists have specialist knowledge of anatomy and biomechanics, physiology and pathology and use the detailed assessment to tailor treatments to each animal, his condition and the stage of the problem.

Members of the Association of Chartered Physiotherapists in Animal Therapy (ACPAT) are chartered physiotherapists who have trained in human physiotherapy and worked in practice before undergoing further training to work with animals. The considerable experience gained in the human field develops skills that are largely transferable to animal physiotherapy. Their experience and specialties are diverse and therefore treatment programmes may be highly specialised.

All chartered physiotherapists abide by the standards for fitness to practice set by the Health Professions Council (HPC) and the Rules of Professional Conduct set by the Chartered Society of Physiotherapy (CSP). This ensures they adhere to the highest standards of health and safety, record-keeping, professionalism and competence, and all maintain full public and professional malpractice indemnity.

The Health Professions Council (HPC) protects the titles 'physiotherapist' and 'physical therapist', but states: 'Prefixes such as 'animal', 'equine', 'veterinary' ... show there is no intention to deceive because the prefix clearly indicates that the person concerned does not treat human beings.' This means that there is currently no protection of the titles of 'veterinary physiotherapist' or 'animal physiotherapist'. However, only members of the Chartered Society of Physiotherapy can call themselves 'chartered physiotherapists'.

What is osteopathy?

The answer to this question has been kindly supplied by Alison Tyler, Osteopath, MSc Animal Manipulation (Osteopathic Pathway).

The science of osteopathy teaches that the structure of the body and how it functions are inextricably linked and that each person contains within themselves the resources necessary for health. In other words, the body is an intrinsically self-healing, self-regulating, self-adjusting organism. Osteopathic treatment works by encouraging the self-healing mechanisms of the body. The primary osteopathic tool, both in assessment and treatment, is the highly skilled sense of touch of the osteopath's hands, known as palpation. During their training osteopaths develop their sense of touch to be able to feel information that is not readily experienced by the untrained hand. With this palpatory skill, applied with a light touch, and a knowledge of anatomy, the osteopath can assess joint mobility and tissue tension and quality, sometimes deep within the body. Osteopathic treatment is designed to break down any compensations and reduce musculoskeletal dysfunction using a variety of different, manual methods including soft tissue massage, mobilisation, manipulation, functional and cranial osteopathic techniques.

The title 'osteopath' is protected, and can only be used by members of the General Osteopathic Council.

What is chiropractic?

The answer to this question has been kindly supplied by Juliet Lock, veterinary chiropractor.

An animal's spine is a complex structure consisting of bones, ligaments, muscles and nerves. Numerous muscles are attached to the vertebrae, enabling the spine to move. Coming out between the vertebrae are pairs of nerves from the spinal cord. Nerves tell the body what to do on a conscious and subconscious level. Nothing can function without a nerve supply. Every movement, from a slight swish of the tail to the complicated one-time changes in dressage, are made possible by synchronising many muscles, which can only function with a nerve supply. Therefore, if there is a restriction within a vertebra, the nerve supply is compromised, which may be painful, and the muscle is less able to function and so performance is reduced. Chiropractors are interested in the restriction of the joints and the resulting impact it can have on the nerves and surrounding tissue. Joints that are slightly restricted tend to cause a loss of performance; joints that are greatly restricted tend to lead to pain.

The title 'chiropractor' is protected, and can only be used by members of the General Chiropractic Council.

15. Where can I find more answers?

If you have other questions, please feel free to contact me through www.holistichorsehelp.com. You can also learn how to massage your horse through the *Horse Massage for Horse Owners* DVD (available from www.holistichorsehelp.com), or through arranging a personal or group Horse Massage for Horse Owners course with me at your yard or at a venue near you.

Prompt Section for Massage Routine

USE THE DIAGRAM AND NOTES here as a reminder of the routine that I've described in Chapter 3. (Swap hands when you swap sides.) To receive a laminated A4 version of this 'prompt sheet' to pin up in your stable yard, simply email your postal address to sue@holistichorsehelp.com and I'll send you a copy.

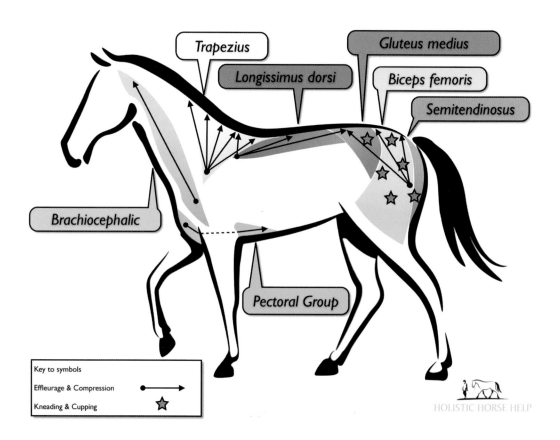

The massage routine reminder

1. Whole body
Stroke horse all over body, taking time to find calm place in your mind.

2. Neck: effleurage x3 on left side of horse.
Apply effleurage with left hand from shoulder to poll (four seconds) then slide hand back to shoulder (four seconds).

3. Neck: compressions x3 on left side of horse.
Slide left hand to poll, then compress between four and ten times, returning from poll to shoulder (each compression taking around four seconds, and stretching the skin away from you).

4. Neck: effleurage x3 on left side of horse.
 As in step two.

5. Repeat steps two to four on right side of horse.

6. Shoulder: effleurage x3 on left side of horse.
Apply effleurage with both hands from beginning to end of outside lines (four seconds) then slide hands back to starting point (four seconds). Repeat along middle lines, and then the inner line, with both hands working together in harmony.

7. Shoulder: compressions x3 on left side of horse.
Slide both hands to end of outside lines (four seconds) then compress between four and ten times (each compression taking around four seconds and stretching the skin away from you) returning to starting point. Repeat along middle lines, then inner line, with both hands working together in harmony.

8. Shoulder: effleurage x3 on left side of horse.
As in step six.

9. Repeat steps five to seven on right side of horse.

10. Back: effleurage x3 on left side of horse.

Apply effleurage using right hand along first line (four seconds), then slide hand back to starting point (four seconds). Repeat along second and third lines.

11. Back: compressions x3 on left side of horse.

Slide right hand to end of line one (four seconds), then compress between four and ten times whilst returning to starting point (each compression taking around four seconds and stretching the skin away from you). Repeat along lines two and three.

12. Back: effleurage x3 on left side of horse.

As in step ten.

13. Repeat steps ten to twelve on right side of horse.

14. Quarters: effleurage x3 on left side of horse

Apply effleurage using right hand from horse's hip along line one (four seconds) then slide hand back to hip (four seconds). Repeat along lines two and three.

15. Quarters: kneading one minute on left side of horse.

Knead with right hand anywhere on the quarters for approximately one minute (each kneading technique taking around four seconds).

16. Quarters: cupping thirty seconds on left side of horse.

Cup with both hands alternately anywhere on quarters for approximately thirty seconds in steady rhythm.

17. Quarters: effleurage x3 on left side of horse.

As in step 14.

18. Repeat steps 14 to 17 on right side of horse.

19. Chest: effleurage x3 on left side of horse.

Apply effleurage from front of horse's chest, between forelegs and towards stomach, starting with left hand and swapping to right hand.

20. Repeat step 19 on right side of horse.

21. Whole body.
Stroke horse all over body as in step one.

22. Thank horse.
Place hand gently on forehead or neck.

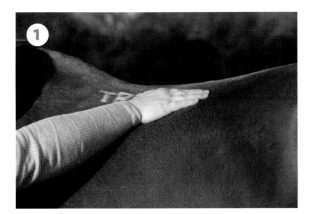

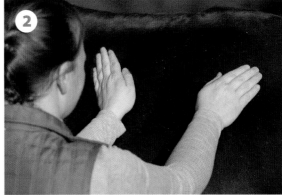

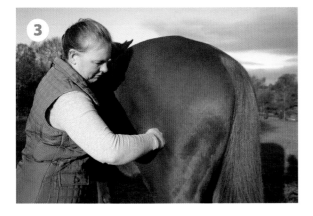

1. Effleurage:
using whole of palm, keep fingers relaxed, always keep contact with horse's skin.

2. Compression:
using heel of hand, squash muscle, stretch skin, release pressure, slide to next spot.

3. Kneading:
using flat of fist, squash muscle, twist skin, release pressure, slide to next spot.

4. Cupping:
using cupped hands, alternately tap muscle.

Useful Information

Below are various sources of further information on topics related to the main text.

Holistic Horse Help
Supporting you towards achieving your dreams with your horse. Founded by Sue Palmer MCSP, MSc Chartered Veterinary Physiotherapist, BHSAI, Equinology Equine Body Worker and Equine Behavioural Consultant. For more information visit www.holistichorsehelp.com

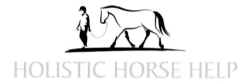

The Association of Chartered Physiotherapy in Animal Therapy (ACPAT)
The professionals in animal therapy. ACPAT is a professional network group of the Chartered Society of Physiotherapy and represents the interests of its members. For more information and to find your local practitioner visit www.acpat.co.uk

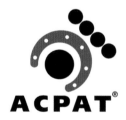

Equinology
Excellent education in equine sports massage, complementary modalities and health. For more information and to find your local practitioner visit

www.equinology.com (Main office, USA, Australia and New Zealand);
www.equinenergy.com (UK and EU);
www.equiworksa.co.za (South Africa) or
www.hoofnpaws.ca (Canada).

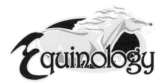

Intelligent Horsemanship

With her mentor Monty Roberts, Kelly Marks promotes respect
and understanding of horses, offering courses, demonstrations and
educational materials. In this effort, the work of the Intelligent
Horsemanship Recommended Associates is also proving to be of
great benefit to horse owners and equine rescue centres. For more
information and to find your local practitioner visit
www.intelligenthorsemanship.co.uk

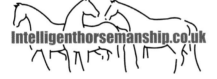

Horse Massage for Horse Owners DVD

'Absolutely HIGHLY recommended – Clear, concise, easy to follow DVD.'
(Review on Amazon). Available from www.holistichorsehelp.com

Into The Lens

Created by Simon Palmer to provide outstanding photographic works
and film footage of the animal world. For more information visit
www.into-the-lens.com

Index